SWALLOW SAFELY

HOW SWALLOWING PROBLEMS THREATEN THE ELDERLY AND OTHERS. A CAREGIVER'S GUIDE TO RECOGNITION, TREATMENT, AND PREVENTION

Roya Sayadi, Ph.D., CCC-SLP

and

Joel Herskowitz, M.D.

INSIDE/OUTSIDE PRESS

Organizations and businesses that deal with elderly persons and
those with particular medical or neurologic disorders are
invited to contact the publisher for information
as to discounts for bulk purchases.

Inside/Outside Press, LLC
P.O. Box 661
Natick, Massachusetts 01760
www.swallowsafely.com
swallowsafely@aol.com

Cover design by Mike Powless of OLM Designs and
Julio Pompa Frizza of Monkey C Media.
Book design by Arrow Graphics, Inc.

Publisher's Cataloging-in-Publication
(Provided by Quality Books, Inc.)

Sayadi, Roya.
    Swallow safely : how swallowing problems threaten the
elderly and others : a caregiver's guide to recognition,
treatment, and prevention / Roya Sayadi and Joel Herskowitz.
    p. cm.
    Includes bibliographical references and index.
    "Help for persons with stroke, Parkinson disease,
multiple sclerosis, Alzheimer disease, ALS, cancer, COPD,
heart disease, and head injury."
    ISBN-13: 978-0-9819601-2-8
    ISBN-10: 0-9819601-2-X

    1. Deglutition disorders--Popular works. 2. Older
people--Care. I. Herskowitz, Joel. II. Title.

RC815.2.S39 2009   616.3'23
                               QBI09-200033

"Don't wait for a swallowing disaster. This book tells you how to keep a swallowing problem from becoming fatal."

—Henry J. Heimlich, M.D.
Author of *Heimlich's Maneuvers*
1984 Recipient of Albert Lasker Public Service Award

"An extremely useful and potentially life-saving book."

—Christiane Northrup, M.D.
Author of *Mother-Daughter Wisdom:*
Understanding the Crucial Link Between
Mothers, Daughters, and Health

"What an eye-opener! Who knew a runny nose could actually be a clue to having a life-threatening swallowing problem? Easy to read and packed with lifesaving knowledge everyone should know. Especially valuable for families and caregivers of elders with dementia, who often develop swallowing problems."

—Jacqueline Marcell
Author of *Elder Rage*
Host of *Coping with Caregiving* on wsRadio.com

"A must-read for seniors and their caregivers. Should be in the library and on the reading list of every senior center in the country!"

—Eric Andersen
CEO and Co-Founder
MySeniorCenter.com

"Swallowing problems often follow severe head trauma. Treating them is a key part of the rehabilitation process. *Swallow Safely* will help save lives by giving family members and other caregivers insight into what can go wrong and what to do about it."

—Dixie Fremont-Smith Coskie
Author of *Unthinkable: A Mother's Tragedy,*
Terror, and Triumph Through a Child's
Traumatic Brain Injury

"Drs. Roya Sayadi and Joel Herskowitz have shown compassion and responsiveness to an important need of our seniors—safety in swallowing. This book is a treasure."

—Betty Perkins-Carpenter, Ph.D.
President, Senior Fitness Productions, Inc.
Author of *How To Prevent Falls*

"I didn't know I had a swallowing problem until I read this book."

—Irwin H. Herskowitz, Ph.D.
Professor Emeritus of Biology (Genetics)
Hunter College, City University of New York

"For people affected neurologically by disorders such as Wilson disease or Parkinson disease, swallowing problems are common and often serious. This book is written for the layperson and provides a much-needed guide for patients and their families or caregivers."

—Carol Terry
Co-Founder, Past President, and Secretary
Wilson Disease Association

"For persons with head and neck cancer, for elderly persons in general, this book will help patients and their families understand and deal with swallowing problems."

—Catherine Thibeault, RN, MSN, MPH
Staff Nurse, Milford Regional Medical Center
Milford, Massachusetts

"Medica Roya Sayadi et Medicus Joel Herskowitz scripserunt librum de morbo gluttiendi qui est tam astutus tam gravis quam Merckus Libellus—sed multo iocior legere." *

—Marian Sniffen
Joel Herskowitz's Latin Teacher at
University City (MO) High School

* "Drs. Roya Sayadi and Joel Herskowitz have written a book about maladies of swallowing that is as knowing and as serious as the Merck Manual—but much more fun to read."

NOTE TO THE READER

This book is intended to provide information for those who wish to learn more about swallowing, related problems, prevention, and treatment. It is in no way intended to replace or to be a substitute for the judgment of a personal treating physician, speech-language pathologist, or other specialist for the diagnosis, treatment, or ongoing care of a patient who has or might have a swallowing problem. The information and opinions provided in this book are believed to be accurate and sound. The reader should consult his or her treating professionals before adopting any of the suggestions in this book.

Recognizing different approaches to the emergency treatment of the conscious choking adult, the publisher and the authors have presented—by means of text and illustrations—principles and practices that are consistent with the highest standards of emergency care. For definitive, up-to-the-minute instruction, the reader is referred to the American Heart Association, the American Red Cross, or a certified CPR instructor.

Neither the publisher nor the authors shall have liability or responsibility to any person or entity with respect to any loss, damage, or injury caused, or alleged to have been caused, directly or indirectly, by the use or application of any of the material contained in this book.

Dedication

To our parents

Farideh Zia
Reza Sayadi
Reida Postrel Herskowitz
Irwin H. Herskowitz

CONTENTS

ILLUSTRATIONS

SUMMARIES

———————

ABOUT THE AUTHORS

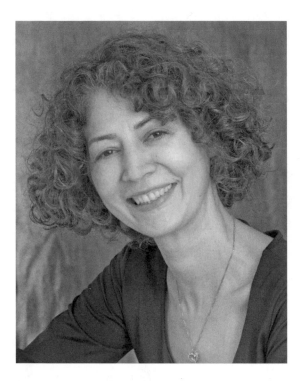

Roya Sayadi, Ph.D., CCC-SLP, is a graduate of the Iran University of Medical Sciences in Tehran. She received her Ph.D. in neurogenic communication disorders from Michigan State University. She has taught speech-language-swallowing pathology at the undergraduate and graduate school levels. She works with the Natick Visiting Nurse Association and has extensive contact with persons who have swallowing problems associated with a wide variety of medical and neurologic illnesses. She lives in Natick, Mass., with her husband. They have four children.

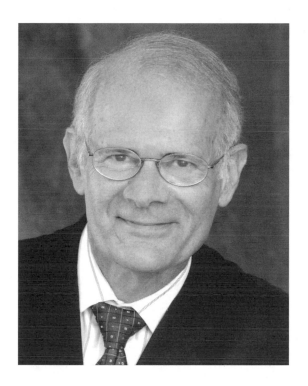

Joel Herskowitz, M.D., Dr. Sayadi's husband, is a graduate of Princeton University and the Albert Einstein College of Medicine. A board-certified pediatric neurologist, he is on the faculty of the Boston University School of Medicine. He is the author of *Pediatrics, Neurology, and Psychiatry: Common Ground* (with N. Paul Rosman, M.D.), *Is Your Child Depressed?*, and *TWISTED!*, a play about a woman with Wilson disease, which he has presented in Boston, Chicago, St. Louis, and Heidelberg, Germany.

Photographs by John Mottern

ACKNOWLEDGMENTS

As a student of speech-language pathology, everything I learned about swallowing, I learned from Jeri Logemann. A professor at Northwestern University and its School of Medicine, Dr. Logemann is a towering figure in the field of speech-language pathology. I came under her influence through her classic textbook, *Evaluation and Treatment of Swallowing Disorders*, as a graduate student at Eastern Michigan and Michigan State Universities, through periodicals she edited, and through conferences she led. Her influence extends to the present. (R.S.)

We thank my father, Irwin H. Herskowitz, Ph.D., and my mother, Reida Postrel Herskowitz, for their critical and helpful reviews of the manuscript; Barrie S. Greiff, M.D., author, psychiatrist, and friend, for his encouragement and suggestions; Henry J. Heimlich, M.D., for his review of portions of the manuscript; Anet James, for her superb illustrations; John Mottern for his photographic contributions; D.J. Hill for her timely and excellent editing; and my sister, Mara Herskowitz, R.N., for allowing us to use a picture of hers for the cover. (J.H.)

Lastly, we acknowledge the contribution of Jamie McDonough, a young man who, in bravely facing the challenges of Wilson disease, made us feel that this book can serve a real purpose not just for the elderly, but for persons of any age whose neurologic disorder or medical condition affects their swallowing.

Roya Sayadi and Joel Herskowitz
Natick, Massachusetts, April 2010

CHAPTER 1

WHY WE WROTE
THIS BOOK

WHY WE WROTE
THIS BOOK

Many people these days know about the dangers of falling in the elderly. A hip fracture, a head injury—a funeral. Falls account for nearly 20,000 deaths per year in this country.

Doctors preach about fall prevention. Magazine articles and books are devoted to the subject. Caregivers are on the alert.

You do many things to reduce the risk of falling in an elderly loved one. You get rid of throw rugs that slip, provide handholds in the bathroom, keep living spaces well lit, watch out for medications that can cause lightheadedness, and promote strength and balance through exercise.

The payoff is greater safety, independence, and peace of mind—theirs and yours.

Swallowing and the Elderly

Did you know that *swallowing problems* are another major threat to the elderly? They, too, account for tens of thousands of deaths in the United States every year. More, perhaps, than falls.

- **Choking** takes nearly four thousand lives.

- **Aspiration** of food, liquid, or bacteria-laden mouth contents into the lungs causes fatal pneumonia in tens of thousands.

- **Malnutrition** resulting from swallowing problems causes weakness and susceptibility to infection that hasten the death of thousands more.

A Vulnerable Population

Nearly 40 million Americans in a total U.S. population of just over 300 million are elderly (65 years of age and older). *From 15 to 50 percent of the elderly are estimated to have a swallowing problem.* That's somewhere between six and 20 million people—and growing.

Swallowing problems account for billions of dollars annually as a result of diagnostic tests, hospitalization, and aftercare costs such as rehabilitation centers, nursing homes, and home-care services. Add to that out-of-pocket and work-related expenses incurred by families involved in caregiving.

So, in terms of lives lost, dollars spent, and schedules disrupted, swallowing problems are no small matter. They are huge.

Has This Happened To You?

When you sit down to dinner with your mother, do you wonder why she constantly clears her throat?

Are you puzzled as to why her nose runs after nearly every meal?

When you give your father juice, do you hold your breath waiting to see if it goes down the right tube?

When he eats a sandwich, are you on the edge of your seat ready to perform the Heimlich maneuver?

Are you forever looking at the kitchen clock when you eat with your mother because meals take so long and you've got a million things to do?

Do you wonder how your loved one can possibly be getting enough food or liquid to survive?

If you've had any of these concerns, you're probably facing significant swallowing issues.

How This Book Came About

This book came about because Roya, a speech-language pathologist with the Visiting Nurse Association based in our hometown of Natick, Massachusetts, was seeing patient after patient with swallowing problems.

These patients—not all elderly—had a wide variety of medical and neurologic disorders: stroke, Alzheimer disease, congestive heart failure, multiple sclerosis, Parkinson disease, ALS (Lou Gehrig's disease), cancer, COPD (chronic obstructive pulmonary disease), diabetes, and head injury. *They all had swallowing problems!*

Typical Scenarios

A 72-year-old man with *Parkinson disease* did everything slowly. Not only were his arms and legs involved, his tongue was, too. So he had difficulty chewing, moving food along, and finally swallowing. Food often got stuck in his throat and caused him to cough and gag.

A 65-year-old woman with a recent *stroke* had difficulty drinking liquids compared with swallowing solid foods. Liquids rushed ahead to cause fits of coughing that brought tears to her eyes. A bout of pneumonia put her back into the hospital and delayed her neurologic recovery.

An 82-year-old man with *Alzheimer disease* required continuous monitoring and assistance with feeding. He was extremely distractible and could no longer use a fork or spoon. He had also "forgotten" what to do with food once it was in his mouth. A single swallow could take three minutes or longer. He was always on the verge of dehydration, no doubt contributing to his tendency to fall.

A 56-year-old woman treated for *salivary gland cancer* had an extremely dry mouth and exquisitely painful sores inside her cheeks. Chewing was painful and her lack of saliva made it difficult to "glue together" a ball of food suitable for swallowing. Eating was altogether unpleasant and left her feeling drained physically and emotionally.

A 49-year-old man with *multiple sclerosis* was able to chew. But when it came to the actual swallow, some of the food was left behind in his throat. It got sucked into his airway; and, because his cough was so weak, the material made its way to his lungs to cause pneumonia.

A typical patient of Roya's had more than one health condition. Parkinson disease, COPD, and diabetes in the same person would not be unusual. Also typical would be for a patient to be taking a dozen medications every day. Their side effects (notably dry mouth) sometimes themselves caused difficulty swallowing.

For a variety of reasons, these patients often did not understand their swallowing problems. As a result, they balked at treatment recommendations or followed them inconsistently, putting themselves in danger.

Their family members, too—trying their best to care for an ill parent, spouse, or adult child—often did not fully appreciate how serious the swallowing problem was. So their ability to support and implement the treatment plan suffered.

A Little Knowledge....Can Be Life-Saving!

Recognizing this knowledge gap, we wanted to write a book that would educate and empower patients and their caregivers.

We have written this book to

- give you a basic understanding of swallowing
- show you how things can go wrong
- explain why swallowing problems are serious
- tell you how to recognize swallowing problems before they become life-threatening
- explain how medications can cause or complicate swallowing problems, and

- guide you in pulling together your observations, questions, and concerns to get help for your loved one.

This book is not intended to be an exhaustive treatment of swallowing problems. Nor is it intended to be a substitute for hands-on evaluation, diagnosis, and treatment by a physician or other qualified swallowing specialist.

Our **Notes** and **Additional Readings** will allow you to delve more deeply into areas of interest. Our **Resources** section and website—**www.swallowsafely.com**—can put you in touch with others who share your concerns.

A Much-Feared Problem

Choking to death can be a caregiver's worst nightmare. If you've sat down to eat with a friend or relative and felt like saying a prayer every time they swallowed, you know what we mean.

It doesn't have to be that way. We explain by word and illustration how choking occurs. We tell you how to reduce the risk of choking and what to do if it happens to another person—or to you.

Crucial Decisions

Because swallowing is vital to nutrition and health, it often becomes a focal point in quality-of-life and end-of-life issues. We believe our book can help elderly patients and their families in making difficult decisions by giving them a better understanding of swallowing problems and treatment options.

Having cared for close family members with swallowing problems related to stroke and cancer, we too have experienced first-hand some of the challenges you're facing.

What's Your Swallowing Story?

We have been struck that almost everyone we meet has a swallowing story. People tell us about an elderly aunt who feared that *choking*, not cancer, would kill her.

They also tell us how they were eating carelessly at a banquet and found themselves on the receiving end of a Heimlich maneuver that saved their life.

Swallow Safely At Any Age

It's not just the elderly who are at risk of swallowing problems. Any adult with medical or neurologic illness—such as lung disease, congestive heart failure, head and neck cancer, stroke, multiple sclerosis, ALS, or Parkinson disease—is vulnerable and will find our discussion of swallowing and its disorders relevant.

We hope, too, that this book will make you more mindful of your own swallowing and prevent problems that could cost you dearly.

And don't forget about your children. Help them establish healthy swallowing habits so that eating and drinking are pleasurable and safe.

Roya's patients and their families tell her: "We didn't realize there was so much to swallowing. We wish we'd known about this sooner."

We believe this book will provide you with useful, potentially-lifesaving information. We wish you the best in helping special persons in your life to **SWALLOW SAFELY**.

CHAPTER 2

HOW SWALLOWING WORKS

How Swallowing Works

Before we look at how things can go wrong, let's look briefly at normal swallowing. The purpose of swallowing is to bring food, liquid, and medication *safely* from the mouth to the stomach.

Normally, swallowing is more than a one-step gulp-and-gone. It's a process. You can use the word "POPE" to remember its four phases:

- Preparatory
- Oral
- Pharyngeal
- Esophageal

1. Preparatory Phase—Forming a Ball of Food

The Preparatory Phase begins even before food gets to your mouth. Your sense of smell—even the anticipation of food—can make your mouth water.

When you take a bite of food, a remarkable dance begins. Your jaws, teeth, cheeks, and tongue work together to make the food into more or less of a ball. This ball of food is called a *bolus* after the Latin word for *ball*.

Your lips close tightly so food doesn't escape from your mouth. Your teeth (or dentures) grind the food into smaller bits. Saliva flows from under and around your tongue. It moistens the food, gathering with it flaky food bits and sugar particles nearby (see Fig. 2-1).

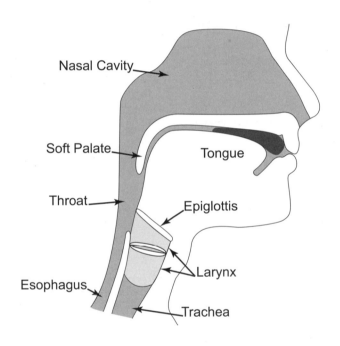

Figure 2-1: Preparatory Phase. Jaws and tongue reduce food to a pasty bolus (in black). (Adapted with permission from *Evaluation and Treatment of Swallowing Disorders, 2nd Ed.*, p. 28, by J.A. Logemann. Copyright 1998 by PRO-ED, Inc., Austin, TX.)

Your tongue mixes and churns the food. It directs the bolus to one side then the other, where your teeth grind it into a dough-like paste. Your jaws move not only up-and-down but in a rotary manner that maximizes grinding.

In addition to physically reducing the mass of solid food, chewing enhances flavor. Juices and other flavorful food elements leak out to contact your taste buds. Enzymes in saliva get to work right away. They start to break down the food while it's still in your mouth.

Your sense of smell gets into the act once again. Aromas pass from throat to nasal cavity where smell receptors enhance the taste of the food and stimulate further saliva flow.

Coordination Required. Just as skilled dancers don't step on each other's toes, we (usually) do not chew on our tongue.

Why not? The tongue sends continuous signals to the brain telling it where the tongue is and what it's doing. Your gums, cheeks, lips, and palate also send information to the brain so you can chew without worrying about chomping on your tongue.

Likewise, breathing and swallowing must work closely together for swallowing to be safe.

Ordinarily, breathing can continue during the Preparatory Phase. But when a medical or neurologic disorder interferes with the balance between the two, breathing and swallowing can become dangerously out of synch.

And, if—under any circumstance—you stir things up further by attempting to swallow while talking, chewing, laughing, *and* breathing, you're asking for trouble. (See Chapters 4 and 5, which discuss *choking* and *aspiration*.)

2. Oral Phase—Transport From Mouth to Throat

Your tongue is now loaded with food. It's like a bucket without a handle. The tongue squeezes the ball of food against the hard palate. This carries the bolus from the front to the back of the mouth, where the *pharynx*, or throat, begins. The entire Oral Phase generally takes about a second (see Fig. 2-2).

The exquisite coordination seen in the Preparatory Phase continues.

- Your lips remain closed to prevent food or liquid from escaping from the front of your mouth.
- Your cheeks stiffen and press against your gums and teeth, which keep food from falling into pockets between cheek and gum.
- Your tongue presses against the bony roof of your mouth to form a muscular chute that directs food to the throat.

18

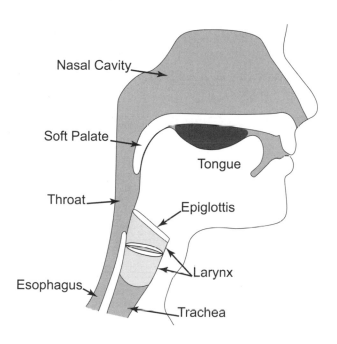

Nasal Cavity

Soft Palate

Tongue

Throat

Epiglottis

Larynx

Esophagus

Trachea

Figure 2-2: Oral Phase. The bolus (in black) is brought from the front to the back of the mouth. (Adapted with permission from *Evaluation and Treatment of Swallowing Disorders, 2nd Ed.*, p. 28, by J.A. Logemann. Copyright 1998 by PRO-ED, Inc., Austin, TX.)

3. Pharyngeal Phase—Pushing It Down

The highlight of the Pharyngeal Phase is the *swallowing reflex*. You could call it the climax of swallowing.

The swallowing reflex is activated by food or liquid reaching the pharynx (see Fig. 2-3). Its entrance is marked by the fleshy pillars that frame the tonsils. This reflex coordinates the many muscles required to push the food down into the esophagus while acting as a safety net to keep it from going where it doesn't belong: the respiratory tract.

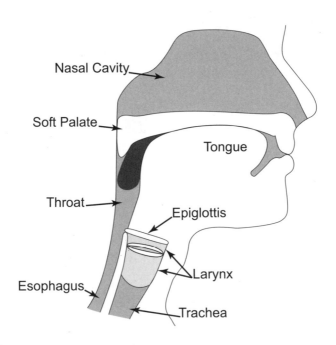

Figure 2-3: Pharyngeal Phase. The bolus (in black) reaches the pharynx to trigger the swallowing reflex. Note the protective changes in position of the soft palate and the epiglottis. (Adapted with permission from *Evaluation and Treatment of Swallowing Disorders*, 2nd *Ed.*, p. 28, by J.A. Logemann. Copyright 1998 by PRO-ED, Inc., Austin, TX.)

Chapter 2: How Swallowing Works

Six hundred or so swallows a day. That's a big job. Without conscious direction, the swallowing reflex weaves together many elements so you can swallow safely.

1. Breathing stops briefly.

2. The tongue and soft palate seal off the roof of the mouth so food doesn't escape through the nose.

3. The hinge-like epiglottis closes over the entrance to the *larynx*, or voice box, which keeps food or liquid from entering the respiratory tract.

4. The larynx moves forward and upward, opening the upper esophagus and further preventing food from getting to the lungs.

5. Within the larynx, the vocal cords come together to keep food or liquid from entering the trachea, or windpipe.

6. Muscles of the pharynx and tongue contract to move the bolus to and through the upper part of the esophagus.

7. The *upper esophageal sphincter* (UES), a ring-shaped muscle at the uppermost esophagus, relaxes to permit food to pass from throat to esophagus (see Figs. 2-4 and 2-5).

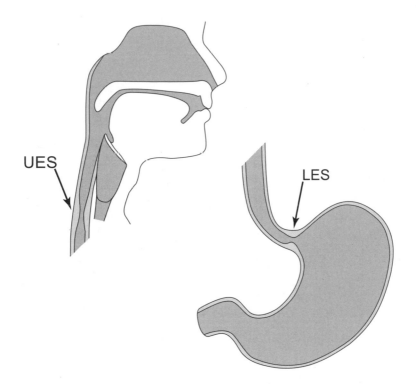

Figure 2-4: Esophageal Sphincters. Food enters the esophagus through the upper esophageal sphinct*er* (UES) and enters the stomach through the lower esophageal sphincter (LES).

The entire Pharyngeal Phase normally takes a second or less. Breathing resumes after the swallow.

A word or two about gagging and vomiting. While the swallowing reflex invites food *in*, gagging and vomiting reflexively send it *out*. A brisk gag does not mean a person has a normal swallow.

4. Esophageal Phase—Getting to the Stomach

Once the bolus gets past the upper esophageal sphincter, this muscular structure contracts tightly to guard against backflow (see Figs. 2-4 and 2-5).

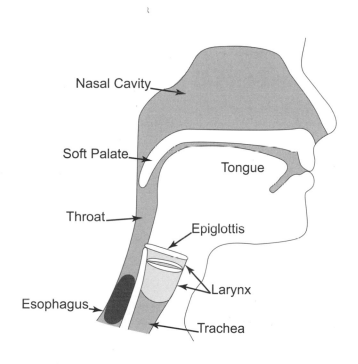

Figure 2-5: Esophageal Phase. The bolus (in black) leaves the pharynx en route to the stomach. (Adapted with permission from *Evaluation and Treatment of Swallowing Disorders, 2nd Ed.*, p. 28, by J.A. Logemann. Copyright 1998 by PRO-ED, Inc., Austin, TX.)

The bolus works its way through the esophagus, moved along by waves of rhythmic contraction (called "peristalsis") to reach the *lower esophageal sphincter* (see Fig. 2-4). Like its upper counterpart, the lower esophageal sphincter is closed at rest. So it must relax to let food pass into the stomach. The entire trip through the esophagus normally takes from eight to twenty seconds.

Phases of Swallowing

1. Preparatory	Forming a ball of food	
2. Oral	Bringing it from mouth to throat	
3. Pharyngeal	Pushing the food down safely	
4. Esophageal	Getting food to the stomach	

Putting It All Together

Let's go for a swallowing walk-through.

Tear off a piece of warm, crusty, freshly baked bread. Hold it in front of you and look at it. Your saliva flows as you prepare for the food to enter your mouth.

The bread passes your lips, and you bite off a hunk. Your tongue greets it and mixes it with saliva, gathering up bits of flaky crust so you don't inhale them. It moves the food to the side where your teeth begin to chew.

Your jaws move up and down, side to side. This rotary action grinds the bolus until it becomes pasty. You continue to breathe while you chew. Your tongue gathers the bolus into a central valley in your mouth, then presses it against the bony palate. Your lips continue their tight seal as your cheeks stiffen further, held closely against your teeth and gums.

The food is brought to the back of the mouth where muscles of the throat and palate block escape through the nasal cavity. The bolus enters the pharynx. Now comes the moment of truth—the swallow itself.

Like a track athlete getting ready for a jump, you pause, gather energy, and hold your breath. Your tongue and throat muscles forcefully contract. Your Adam's apple rises as your larynx elevates and squeezes tightly shut, closing off the airway. You swallow. The food leaves your throat to begin its downward descent. You release air through your nose as you resume breathing.

Your tongue searches out remnants of food that may have been left between gum and cheek. You swallow one or several times more to finish things off, perhaps clearing your throat between swallows. The final swallow is little more than saliva.

You can turn this thought exercise into a real-life experience by getting a piece of bread or chunk of apple and observing yourself as you chew and swallow.

Are you able to follow the various phases? Do you see how active the tongue is in its many roles? Making food into a ball? Positioning it for chewing? Bringing it to the back of the mouth? Pushing it down? Cleaning up afterwards? Did you notice how breathing stops during the swallow?

We think you'll agree—there's a lot going on here. Swallowing is a complicated process, something we generally take for granted when all is well. In the next chapter, we look at how swallowing can break down.

CHAPTER 3

WHEN SWALLOWING DOESN'T WORK

WHEN SWALLOWING DOESN'T WORK

Now that we've looked at normal swallowing phase by phase, you have a framework for understanding how things can go wrong.

Before going any further, we need to define an important word: *dysphagia* (pronounced "diss-FAY-juh"). Simply put, dysphagia means "difficulty swallowing."

Difficulty swallowing is always of concern. It can put a person at risk of choking and aspiration, interfere with proper nutrition, and make meals anxiety-provoking, time-consuming, and frustrating.

What Dysphagia Feels Like

These are some of the things people complain of when they have difficulty swallowing:

"The food doesn't go down."

"I have to swallow more than once."

"Tears come to my eyes when I eat."

"My nose runs at mealtimes."

"Pills get stuck in my throat."

29

"I cough when I drink water."

"The food falls out of my mouth."

"I have a hard time eating steak."

"When I swallow, juice goes up my nose."

"It hurts when I swallow."

"I'm afraid I'm going to choke."

"My voice sounds funny after I eat."

"I get so tired, I can't finish a meal."

"What do you expect? I'm old."

Sometimes, a person has no complaint at all—but a very real problem with swallowing.

Where Swallowing Breaks Down

Swallowing problems can arise at any step in the swallowing process (Fig. 3-1). They can result from structural, neurologic, or general causes.

- *Structural* refers to anatomy. Something is missing (due to birth defect, injury, or surgery) or extra (such as a cancerous tumor, cyst, diverticulum, or aneurysm).

- *Neurologic* refers to a disease process that interferes with muscle control, speed, or coordination (as with Parkinson disease, stroke, multiple sclerosis, or ALS).

- *General* refers to a condition that causes overall weakness (such as congestive heart failure or COPD).

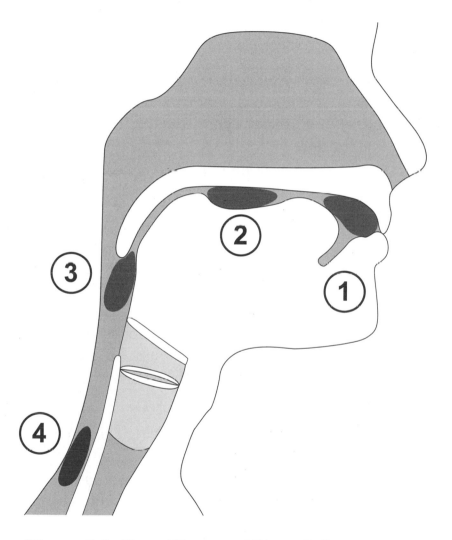

Figure 3-1: Four Phases of Normal Swallowing.
(1) Preparatory, (2) Oral, (3) Pharyngeal,
(4) Esophageal.

1. Preparatory Phase Problems

As we have seen, a good supply of saliva helps to make a well-chewed, pasty bolus that slides safely through the throat and esophagus. Saliva acts like glue in holding together the various foodstuffs that are combined to form a cohesive bolus.

Cut down on your saliva flow (through dehydration, drug effect, or Sjögren's syndrome, for example) and you can interfere with any phase of swallowing. This can be the tipping point for a serious swallowing problem.

Losing one's sense of smell or taste can also reduce the supply of saliva. This can be caused by infections of the nose, mouth, or throat; tobacco use; allergies; dental disease; diabetes; underactive thyroid; medications (see Chapter 6); Parkinson disease; Alzheimer disease; Huntington disease; multiple sclerosis; brain tumor; vitamin or mineral deficiency (including B12 or zinc); radiotherapy; chemotherapy; Sjögren's syndrome; and old age.

Keep in mind that anything blocking the sense of smell will also interfere with taste sensation. Furthermore, a medication might not *abolish* the sense of taste but *alter* it, for example, making some foods taste "metallic."

Swallowing and Dehydration. Dehydration is caused by too little water coming in, too much water going out, or both. A person who is dehydrated will cry fewer tears, urinate less often, and produce less saliva.

Causes of Dehydration

- A lack of thirst commonly occurs with Alzheimer disease, stroke, brain tumor, head trauma, and old age.

- Some people might avoid going to the kitchen or bathroom for a drink of water because weakness, dizziness, or loss of balance makes it difficult or dangerous to do so.

- Neurologic disorders such as Parkinson disease, Alzheimer disease, and ALS can slow down eating and drinking to such a degree that it becomes virtually impossible for a person to take in adequate food or liquid by mouth.

- Depressed persons often lose their appetite for drink as well as for food. Antidepressant medication can make matters worse by causing dry mouth (see Chapter 6).

- Excessive water loss from sweating may result from environmental causes. The thermostat is set too high. The air conditioner is not working. A person is under too many blankets.

- The nearly continuous muscle activity that can occur with dystonia, Wilson disease, and some forms of cerebral palsy can similarly cause a tremendous amount of water loss due to sweating.

- Increased urination with *diabetes mellitus* ("sugar diabetes"), *diabetes insipidus* (following head trauma or with renal disease), or *diuretic medication* (used to treat congestive heart failure or high blood pressure) can lead to dehydration.

- Vomiting, diarrhea, or fever of any cause can cause dehydration as well.

It's not just swallowing that suffers when you're dehydrated. Dehydration also means less blood to the brain and muscles. That can interfere with thinking, balance, and overall strength—making a person confused, dizzy, and weak. Plus, a dehydrated person often feels just plain miserable!

Effects of Cancer Treatment. Radiotherapy or chemotherapy can cause dry mouth and cracking of mucous membranes that line the mouth and throat. They can also interfere with a person's immune system, setting the stage for infection with yeast and other germs.

As a result, movements of the lip, cheek, or tongue can become exquisitely painful. This can make chewing and swallowing a torture, creating a vicious cycle of dehydration, malnutrition, and weakness leading to more of the same.

Denture Danger. Poorly fitting dentures—often associated with painful gums—can interfere with chewing and pave the way for major problems. Add impatience, inattentiveness, difficulty cutting with a knife and fork, and a bit of alcohol, and you have a recipe for a choking emergency (see Chapter 4).

Furthermore, dentures (and underlying gums) that are not cleaned regularly are a rich source of bacteria that can get to the lungs to cause pneumonia.

Pulmonary Problems. For a mouth-breather the simple act of swallowing can be a disaster waiting to happen. A poorly timed, gasping breath can suck food or liquid into the lungs to cause pneumonia. Or it may block the airway entirely, presenting an immediate threat to life.

Drinking from a cup can be a particular challenge for persons with respiratory disease. When we drink, we usually take a series of gulps while holding our breath for several seconds.

That brief period without breathing may be more than someone with a respiratory condition can tolerate. It can create sputtering, gasping, and acute distress.

2. Oral Phase Problems

The Oral Phase is all about transport. Having a dry mouth interferes not just with bolus formation but with passage of the bolus through the mouth.

As you know, the tongue plays the key role in bringing food from the front to the back of the mouth, where the swallowing reflex takes over. Anything that affects the structure or function of the tongue will influence swallowing, for example, surgical removal of part of the tongue in cancer treatment.

With neurologic disorders such as Parkinson disease, brainstem stroke, ALS, Wilson disease, and Huntington disease, slow, poorly controlled tongue, lip, and jaw movements interfere with bolus formation and transport. Dehydration, malnutrition, and the threat of choking or aspiration are constant concerns.

The Tongue's Many Roles

Promotes taste and enjoyment of food

Places food in position for chewing

Mixes food with saliva to create bolus

Transports bolus from front to back of mouth

Helps push the food down

Cleans up after the swallow

Swallowing and Stroke. Swallowing problems are a common, potentially life-threatening complication of stroke, accounting for thousands of deaths per year. The type of swallowing problem will depend upon the nature and extent of the stroke: hemispheric or brainstem, motor or sensory.

The good news is that through effective medical care and specific swallowing therapy many persons who have suffered a stroke will be able to resume eating a relatively normal diet within weeks to months.

Paralysis of tongue, lip, and cheek muscles interferes with chewing, transport, swallowing, and cleaning up after the swallow. Food spills out from the front of the mouth. Liquids get to the throat without control or direction, before protective mechanisms are in place. Food left behind can readily be aspirated.

Sensory loss, too, can throw off any phase of swallowing. The brain needs to know what kind of food the mouth is working on, where the bolus is, and whether any food remains after the swallow. When sensation is absent, the swallowing reflex will not be activated.

Loss of sensation can also interfere with coughing. Without an effective cough response, food or liquid that gets into the airway has a free pass to the lungs.

37

3. Pharyngeal Phase Problems

Once food has reached the pharynx, the swallowing reflex is activated. As we saw in Chapter 2, many things come together to ensure that swallowing is accomplished safely.

Because the swallowing reflex is based in the brainstem, neurologic disorders affecting this part of the nervous system will influence the Pharyngeal Phase of swallowing. These include multiple sclerosis, Parkinson disease, ALS, and some types of stroke.

A nasal quality to the voice or regurgitation of liquid through the nose suggests involvement of the brainstem. These result from inadequate closure of the soft palate, a hallmark of ALS.

With myasthenia gravis or muscular dystrophy the muscles may simply become too weak to push the food down. Overall weakness due to heart disease, lung problems, or cancer can have the same effect.

Those who have undergone intubation—placement of a tube into the trachea to support breathing—can later experience swallowing difficulties. Scar tissue resulting from difficult or prolonged intubation can prevent complete closure of the vocal cords during the swallowing reflex, creating a "hole" in the swallowing safety net.

Zenker Diverticulum. Swallowing is a muscular activity. It generates great force within the throat. Not surprisingly, decades of swallowing can weaken the pharynx and cause throat tissue to balloon out or protrude.

Such an outpouching, called a *Zenker diverticulum*, commonly forms where the throat meets the esophagus. As a result, food is waylaid en route to the stomach and hides out in this pouch. That can lead to bad breath, frequent coughing, regurgitation, or worse—choking or aspiration.

4. Esophageal Phase Problems

Food must get *to* the esophagus, then *through* the esophagus. To enter the esophagus, food passes through the upper esophageal sphincter (UES) (see Figs. 2-4 and 2-5). Recall that this sphincter is contracted at rest and relaxes as part of the swallowing reflex to let food through.

With neurologic disorders, formation of scar tissue, or compression by a tumor anywhere within the chest, this sphincter may not open fully. As a result, something less than the entire bolus gets through to the esophagus.

If the upper esophageal sphincter shuts too soon, it pinches off part of the bolus before it enters the esophagus. In either case, food stays in the throat, ready to fall (or to be inhaled) into an unprotected airway.

Achalasia: A Failure To Relax. The lower esophageal sphincter is the gateway to the stomach (see Fig. 2-4). With *achalasia*, this sphincter fails to relax to permit the bolus to enter the stomach.

This creates a backup much like a clogged drainpipe. Persons with achalasia may have difficulty swallowing, a feeling of fullness, chest discomfort, or regurgitation.

Other Esophageal Problems. The esophagus is a favorite target of *scleroderma*, an autoimmune disorder that affects connective tissue. Stiffened esophageal walls or constricting scar tissue can interfere with passage of a bolus. Achalasia and esophagitis—irritation of the esophagus from reflux or infection—also occur commonly with scleroderma.

With *gastroesophageal reflux disease* (GERD), acidic digestive juices flow from the stomach back to the esophagus. Over time, irritation and inflammation of the lining of the esophagus may lead to scarring, stricture formation, and ultimately cancer.

Now that we've looked at swallowing problems phase by phase, let's turn our attention to one of the most feared swallowing problems: *choking*.

Overview of
Causes of Swallowing Difficulty

Preparatory   Loss of smell or taste sensation; lack of saliva; weak chewing muscles; mouth pain; poorly-fitting dentures; lack of tongue control; mouth-breathing

Oral   Part of tongue missing, impaired tongue control, sensory loss

Pharyngeal   Absent or delayed reflex, muscle paralysis or weakness, sensory loss, diverticula, lack of coordination with breathing

Esophageal   Malfunction of upper and lower sphincters (achalasia, GERD); lack of esophageal motility; stiffness, stricture, or compression of esophagus

A *Structural, Neurologic, or General Disease Process Can Act at Any Phase*

CHAPTER 4

WHAT TO DO ABOUT CHOKING

WHAT TO DO
ABOUT CHOKING

The best thing to do about choking is, of course, to keep it from happening. That's a large part of what we're trying to do in this book.

Choking is scary. But it's not just anxiety-provoking. It accounts for thousands of deaths per year—with the elderly at highest risk.

By understanding the basics of swallowing and what can go wrong, you can take steps to reduce the risk of choking.

Unfortunately, it is not always going to be possible to prevent choking. So if you're assisting an elderly loved one at home, dining with friends at a restaurant, or eating by yourself, we want you to be able to recognize a choking emergency and deal with it effectively.

What Is Choking?

In everyday use, *choking* refers to gagging or coughing in response to the feeling that something is stuck. It won't go down. There is often a sense of urgency, a feeling that "It has to come out—or else!"

In this book, we generally use the word *choking* in a narrower sense to mean *airway obstruction*. This refers specifically to (1) blockage of airflow to a person's lungs or (2) the person's behavioral response to such obstruction.

Since our lives depend upon a steady supply of oxygen, a blockage of any kind is important. Complete lack of oxygen causes brain damage after about four minutes and death within around ten.

Food, pills, or non-food objects (such as a bone, piece of chewing gum, or bottle cap) can lodge in the throat to prevent air from getting *to* the airway (see Fig. 4-1).

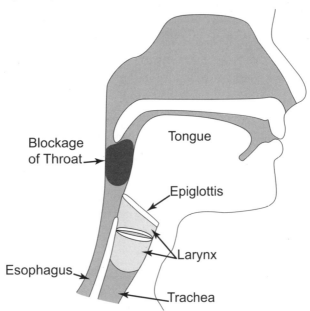

Figure 4-1: Blocking the Throat. An object blocks the throat, preventing air from getting *to* the airway. Or an object gets into the windpipe itself, preventing air from getting *through* the airway (see Fig. 4-2).

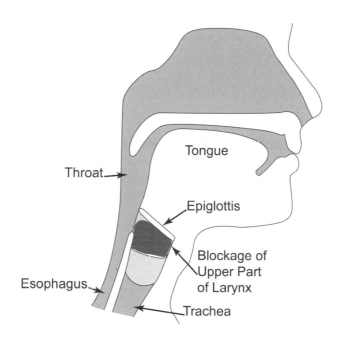

Figure 4-2: Blocking the Trachea. An object has entered the larynx ("voice box"), the uppermost part of the trachea, preventing breathing or talking.

It doesn't take much to block the airway. At its widest part, the larynx is slightly less than two inches in an adult male. The trachea below narrows to around one inch in diameter. So you can see how easily a chunk of hot dog, a piece of steak, or a glob of peanut butter-and-jelly sandwich can fully obstruct the airway.

47

Risk Factors For Choking

The elderly are at highest risk of death by choking, even more so than young children. Several factors make them especially vulnerable.

Why the Elderly are at Increased Risk

- Missing teeth or having ill-fitting dentures
- Having a complicated medical picture
- Having a neurologic disorder
- Taking medications that cause dry mouth, drowsiness, or muscle stiffness

---

Some people don't chew their food at all. Autopsy results have yielded startlingly large pieces of unchewed steak the size of a deck of cards that block the airway.

Congestive heart failure and respiratory illnesses, among other medical conditions, can weaken a person and interfere with a vigorous, protective cough. Side effects of medications can cause or contribute to swallowing difficulties (see Chapter 6).

With Parkinson disease, the whole swallowing process slows down. Coordination between breathing and swallowing is thrown off. Coughing is weak. See Chapter 3 for ways neurologic disorders at any age predispose to choking.

The "Café Coronary"

A person choking on food can look for all the world like he's having a heart attack—especially if he is middle-aged or older.

Unless it is recognized for what it is—a life-threatening choking incident—this "café coronary" can end a life as surely as a bona fide heart attack.

"Coronary" is short for *coronary occlusion* or *thrombosis*, a blockage of coronary vessels that supply blood to the heart. This can cause a heart attack, or *myocardial infarction.*

When you suspect a heart attack, calling for emergency medical help is the right thing to do. But if a person is choking, waiting for an ambulance to arrive without doing anything else may be a fatal mistake.

The café coronary is, of course, not restricted to establishments where you're expected to leave a tip. It can happen at your home or your mother's. So be prepared.

"Café Coronary" vs. Heart Attack
(In a conscious person)

Choking episode . . . . Unable to speak or breathe

Myocardial infarction . . . Able to speak and breathe

A Signal For Action

The choking person may have a *completely* or *partially* blocked airway. Either may require emergency intervention.

When the airway is completely blocked, a person will not be able to breathe, talk, or cough. His face will become gray or blue. His eyes may "bug out" in panic. He may collapse and lose consciousness.

When the airway is partially blocked, the person may be able to breathe—but only with difficulty or perhaps with a wheeze. If she can speak at all, her voice may be high-pitched, strained, noisy, or weak.

The choking person may give a sign of distress—thumb and index finger encircling the neck (see Fig. 4-3). These situations call for action.

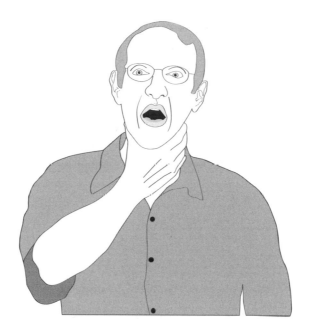

Figure 4-3: Choking Distress Signal. May be accompanied by turning blue, bulging eyes, running away in distress.

Ask the person, "Are you choking?" If he nods his head "Yes" or does not respond, act immediately. *Perform the Heimlich maneuver.*

Do *not* slap him on the back with the hope of dislodging the obstructing material. That could lodge the object more firmly against the airway or deeper into the trachea.

Do *not* reach into the throat to try to remove food. That wastes time and could push the material in further.

51

If the person is able to cough, let him. That can be an effective way of correcting the problem. Hold off on your Heimlich maneuver for the time being.

Watch carefully. If the person is barely able to talk or breathe, get ready to administer the Heimlich maneuver. If you have an emergency alert device, activate it. Call 911 if necessary (for example, if the person collapses).

If a choking person—out of embarrassment or anxiety—leaves the dining area (whether at home or a restaurant) seeking privacy, *you must follow him!* Stay with him until the matter is resolved. A failure to see the incident through could be fatal (see Fig. 4-4).

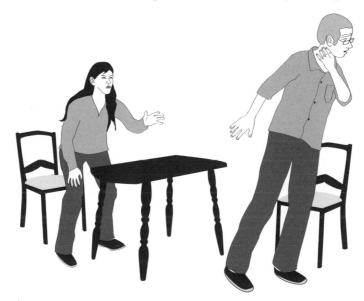

Figure 4-4: Follow That Person! The choking victim may leave the area to avoid embarrassment. Follow and provide emergency treatment as needed.

The Heimlich Maneuver

To perform the Heimlich maneuver, get behind the choking person who is seated or standing. Wrap your arms around her waist. Place the thumb side of one fist against the upper abdomen above the umbilicus (the belly button) just below the sternum (the lowermost ribcage). Wrap your other hand around the pinky side of your fist (see Fig. 4-5).

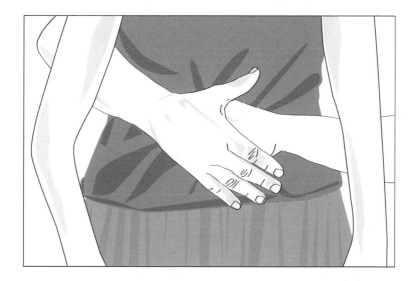

Figure 4-5: Hand Position For Heimlich Maneuver. Place the thumb side of your fist against the choking person's abdomen, between belly button and sternum. Then wrap the fist with your other hand.

With a quick, upward thrust, pull your hands toward yourself against the person's abdomen. You may actually lift the person off the chair or the floor. Repeat several times if necessary (see Fig. 4-6).

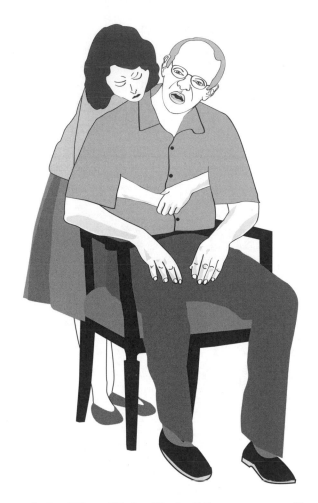

Figure 4-6: The Heimlich Maneuver. Carrying out the maneuver when the choking person is seated.

If the choking person collapses or is too large for you to get your arms around (for example, if a small woman is rescuing a large adult), quickly lay the person down face up.

Get on your knees at the level of the upper thigh or hips and place the heel of your hand just above the umbilicus, below the rib cage. Place your free hand upon the other. Press into the abdomen with quick, forward thrusts. Repeat several times if needed (see Fig. 4-7).

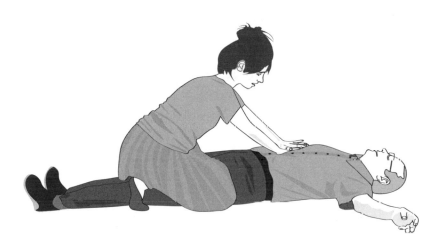

Figure 4-7: Victim on Floor. If the victim has collapsed or is too large, perform the Heimlich maneuver on the floor. Call 911 as soon as possible.

If another person is present, have her remove any food material that has been expelled into the mouth so it doesn't cause further blockage and choking. If the person vomits, turn the entire body to one side to prevent aspiration. Remove the vomited material as quickly as possible.

If two or three attempts do not expel the choking object and restore breathing, continue the procedure and have someone call 911.

There's no harm, of course, if a person on the scene calls 911 sooner rather than later. If you're alone with a choking victim, however, proceed at once to the Heimlich maneuver.

Some sources recommend sharp blows to the back if abdominal thrusts do not work or even before the Heimlich maneuver. We follow the recommendation of the American Heart Association as to clearing a blocked airway in a conscious adult or older child, namely, proceeding directly to the Heimlich maneuver.

Saving Your Own Life

You can choke while eating alone. For that reason, you need to know how to carry out the Heimlich maneuver on yourself.

If you choke and find yourself unable to speak, cough, or breathe, don't panic. If you have an emergency contact device, trigger it immediately. Carry out the Heimlich maneuver without delay.

Stand against a sink, countertop, desk, or sturdy chair. Press your upper belly firmly against its upper edge, grasping its sides with both hands. Thrust yourself forward vigorously, bending slightly at the waist. Repeat as needed (see Fig. 4-8).

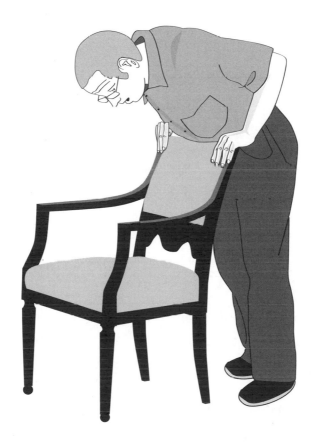

Figure 4-8: The Self-Heimlich Maneuver. Use chair, desk, countertop—or your own fist.

If a desk or other suitable structure is not available, use your own wrapped fist to carry out the abdominal thrusts.

Why The Heimlich Maneuver Works

As Dr. Henry Heimlich explained some 35 years ago, choking is common when a person talks or laughs while swallowing food. The food blocks the larynx (the voice box), which is why a person can't talk or breathe.

By pressing against the upper abdomen, between the umbilicus and the chest, you push the diaphragm upward into the chest, making the chest cavity smaller. This compresses the lungs, causing a strong flow of air out the airway. The air flow carries the obstructing object out of the airway and out of the mouth.

Post-Heimlich Check-Up

We recommend that after you have carried out the Heimlich maneuver on an elderly person you take him for a medical examination to check for complications such as a broken rib or damage to an internal organ.

Keep in mind that the object the person was choking on sometimes gets through to the lungs. Weeks, even months, later she may show symptoms of respiratory illness (such as pneumonia or lung abscess) arising from that incident.

What To Do About Choking

Prevention   Follow safe swallowing strategies

Be prepared for an emergency at all times, especially in persons with medical or neurologic illness

Recognition   Watch for a choking distress signal, inability to breathe or talk, agitation, leaving the room

Action   Follow the person
Observe
Let the person cough
Perform the Heimlich maneuver if necessary
Call 911
Activate emergency alert device

Follow-Up   Carry out post-Heimlich maneuver checkup
Watch for later illness

The next chapter deals with another complication of swallowing difficulty that can have a fatal outcome: *aspiration.*

CHAPTER 5

ASPIRATION AND PNEUMONIA

ASPIRATION AND
PNEUMONIA

Remember the time you were having lunch with a couple of friends. Chatting, laughing, having a pleasant afternoon. All of a sudden you had a violent coughing fit that brought tears to your eyes.

A minute or so later, when the attack subsided and everyone could breathe again, a friend asked: "What happened?"

"I think food went down the wrong tube," you said.

That's the essence of *aspiration*—food, liquid, or other material getting into the wrong tube: the trachea instead of the esophagus (see Fig. 5-1).

Because you were in good health, you got rid of the offending material by means of coughing vigorously. But what about your elderly aunt? She's not in the best of health—weak overall—and her cough is anything but strong.

If something gets into her airway, it has a good chance of getting to her lungs. That could be the ticket to pneumonia, deterioration, and death—a common sequence in persons with Parkinson disease, Alzheimer disease, ALS, and other neurologic disorders.

Aspiration vs. Penetration

Strictly speaking, *aspiration* is defined by material passing beyond the vocal cords, which lie within the larynx, the uppermost part of the trachea. Until that point, it's considered *penetration*. That's probably what happened to you at lunch the other day.

Aspiration can result from problems at any phase of the swallowing process:

- a lack of saliva or weak chewing muscles— anything that prevents formation of a proper bolus (*Preparatory*);

- a tongue under poor control, unable to transport a bolus effectively from mouth to throat (*Oral*);

- lack of coordination between breathing and swallowing; a faulty swallowing reflex with incomplete palatal closure or weak pharyngeal muscles that can't push the food down (*Pharyngeal*);

- a scarred upper esophageal sphincter that doesn't open fully to permit passage of a complete bolus or an incompetent lower esophageal sphincter that allows foodstuff to back up to the throat (*Esophageal*).

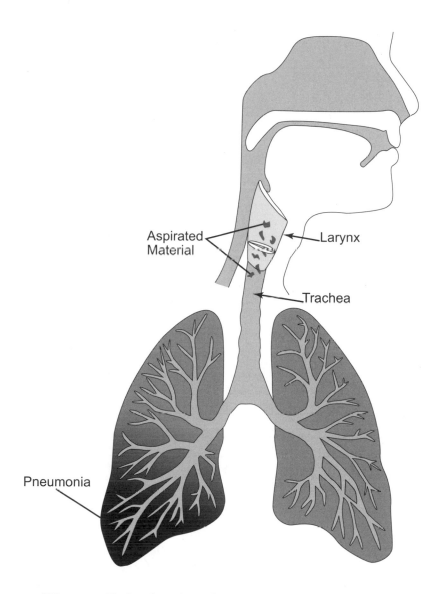

Figure 5-1: Aspiration and Pneumonia. Food, liquid, medication, or other material passes through the larynx and trachea to reach the lungs, where it can cause pneumonia.

Symptoms of Unsafe Swallowing

These signs and symptoms during eating or drinking suggest an unsafe swallow and increased risk of aspiration:

- coughing
- "choking"
- sputtering
- tearing of the eyes
- runny nose (due to increased tearing)
- wheezing
- change in voice after the swallow (weak, hoarse, or gargly)
- needing to swallow more than once
- tired out by eating
- feeling food is stuck in throat
- repeated bouts of pneumonia.

Be aware that aspiration can take place without any warning signs whatsoever, called *silent aspiration*. We'll talk more about that later in this chapter.

You don't have to be elderly to be at risk for aspiration. Also vulnerable are younger people with medical or neurologic illnesses such as congestive heart failure, stroke, Alzheimer disease, Parkinson disease, multiple sclerosis, head trauma, and ALS. Aspiration can, of course, occur at any age due to carelessness.

Aspiration and Pneumonia

Aspiration pneumonia is an inflammatory condition that results from entry of material into the lungs. Material aspirated from the nose, mouth, teeth, dentures, or throat typically contains large numbers of bacteria that can cause an infectious pneumonia. Repeated episodes of aspiration and poor dental hygiene increase the likelihood of pneumonia.

Material aspirated from the stomach or esophagus typically has fewer bacteria but may contain irritating stomach acid. This stomach acid can cause a chemical pneumonia, called *pneumonitis*. This term reflects the irritative nature of the process and differentiates it from *pneumonia*, which generally indicates an infectious origin.

Pneumonitis and pneumonia typically arise in different kinds of clinical situations. *Aspiration pneumonitis* characteristically occurs in persons who have had a sudden and profound change in mental state—for example, with drug overdose, head injury, seizure, or general anesthesia. Pneumonitis results from vomiting with aspiration of acidic stomach contents.

Aspiration pneumonia generally occurs under less acute circumstances. Bacteria-laden material from the nose, throat, gums, or dentures enters the airway through any of a series of mishaps and proceeds to the lungs to cause pneumonia.

67

The terms *pneumonia* and *pneumonitis* are often used interchangeably. Don't let the terminology confuse you. The take-home point in either case is that aspiration has caused a serious lung problem.

Typical symptoms of aspiration pneumonia include rapid, effortful breathing, cough, chest pain, wheezing, and fever. Elderly persons, however, may not have these typical symptoms of respiratory illness. Their pneumonia may declare itself by confusion, delirium, weakness, or falling.

The Cough as Clue

We tend to think of a cough as little more than an annoyance. A scratchy throat. The beginning of a cold. Nothing to worry about.

By now you know that cough may be the sign of a swallowing problem. We're not saying every cough is due to aspiration. What we *are* saying is that chronic cough, unexplained pneumonia, or signs and symptoms listed earlier in this chapter should raise the question of aspiration or other swallowing problem.

An Unsettling Fact—Silent Aspiration

Aspiration does not always cause obvious symptoms. It can be *silent*—without coughing, tearing, wheezing, voice change, or other symptoms.

Silent aspiration can occur while a person is awake

or asleep. It can occur as well in those who receive tube feedings or are on a ventilator.

Even experienced swallowing specialists cannot always diagnose clinically significant aspiration with complete accuracy by observing a person at the bedside or in the office. They must combine the patient's history and clinical examination with specialized tests of swallowing for definitive diagnosis (see Chapter 8).

That's why it's important for caregivers to keep the possibility of aspiration in mind when a loved one has a cough that won't go away or has been treated for pneumonia more than once. If you suspect silent aspiration, bring it up with your doctor or swallowing specialist.

Is *Your* Swallowing Unsafe?

Getting back to that unpleasant experience at lunch—something like this can happen to anyone. If it has happened to you or to a loved one more than once, however, pay close attention.

If you've experienced voice change, wheezing, pneumonia, or other symptoms of respiratory illness after a swallowing incident, consider aspiration as a possibility.

Is there something unsafe about your swallowing? What caused that nasty fit of coughing? Do you eat too quickly? Do you chew your food enough? Were you drinking alcohol? Were you laughing, talking, and trying to swallow at the same time?

Look at your eating habits. Make some changes if you need to. That could save *your* life.

Overview of Aspiration

Definition	Food, drink, or medication going down the wrong tube
Major Complications	Pneumonia; pneumonitis
Symptoms	Coughing, tearing, voice change, wheezing, lung disease, none
Diagnosis	In the office; at the bedside; by special investigation
Prevention and Early Detection	In elderly persons, adults of any age with medical or neurologic disorders, your children, yourself

---

In the next chapter, we explore ways that medications—which are supposed to make things better—can make them *worse*.

CHAPTER 6

MEDICATION:
A DOUBLE-EDGED SWORD

MEDICATION:
A DOUBLE-EDGED SWORD

At times it seems as if the elderly are swimming in a sea of pills!

Let's look at your father. He has four major medical problems: diabetes, Parkinson disease, COPD, and depression. His doctors have him on more than a dozen pills a day. That calls for a lot of organization—*and* a lot of swallowing.

If he has any kind of swallowing difficulty, the chance of something bad happening is multiplied. Some of

How Medications
Cause Swallowing Problems

- Reduce the supply of saliva
- Interfere with smell, taste, and appetite
- Cause drowsiness or inattention
- Irritate the throat or esophagus
- Allow overgrowth of harmful germs
- Cause swallowing muscles to tighten
- Slow passage of food through the esophagus
- Relax the lower esophageal sphincter to allow for reflux

that medication could wind up burning his esophagus or getting sucked into his lungs.

Medications save lives. They help maintain quality of life. But their *side effects* can themselves create swallowing problems.

Increasing the Risk

The sheer number of pills can itself be a challenge. It requires a workable system to ensure that a person doesn't miss taking one medication and double up on another.

The challenge can be physical, too. Taking what seems to be an endless round of pills can be fatiguing, anxiety-provoking, and altogether annoying. The first swallows may be fine—the last ones difficult and dangerous.

When a person takes multiple medications, the potential for side effects is magnified. Drugs are metabolized by the liver and kidneys. When

Multiple Medications: Increased Risks

- Greater likelihood of medication error by patient or doctor
- More opportunity to choke or aspirate
- Increased drug strength
- Prolonged duration of action

medications compete for breakdown and excretion, this can result in elevated blood levels and a longer stay in the body. Either one increases the risk of harmful side effects.

What Does "Anticholinergic" Mean?

When you read about side effects of medication in the elderly, you will soon come across the word *anticholinergic*. It means "acting against *choline*," a shortened form of *acetylcholine*.

Acetylcholine ("uh-SEE-t'l-KOH-leen") is a chemical messenger, a neurotransmitter. Starting out in the brain, it is distributed widely throughout the body.

In the brain, acetylcholine is involved in memory, in the mouth for salivation, in the skin for sweating,

Anticholinergic Side Effects

Dry mouth	Eye pain
Sticky lips	Sensitivity to light
White-coated tongue	Urinary retention
Dehydration	Constipation
Loss of taste	Rapid heart rate
Decreased appetite	Dizziness
Fever	Memory impairment
Red, hot skin	Confusion
Enlarged pupils	Agitation
Blurred vision	

in the bladder for urination, in the eyes for vision, and in the gastrointestinal tract for moving food along. An *anticholinergic* drug thus can have a variety of effects.

Dry mouth can be an especially troublesome anticholinergic side effect. It can make it difficult for pills to pass easily through the mouth, throat, and esophagus. Gelatinous capsules in particular can readily stick to their lining to produce a chemical burn.

Anticholinergic effects are not always negative. Sometimes they're desirable, as in the treatment of urinary incontinence, Parkinson disease, drooling, and irritable bowel syndrome. Belladonna preparations, for example, containing the potent anticholinergic agent atropine, have long been used for treating intestinal cramps and diarrhea.

"Beautiful Lady"

In sixteenth century Italy, women applied a belladonna solution to their eyes to enlarge their pupils. It was felt to make them more attractive, hence, the name *bella donna*, Italian for *beautiful lady*.

Your mother at any age is beautiful. But if her pupils are unusually large, if she complains that light bothers her, if she has blurry vision, or if she has any other of the previously listed side effects (such as a change in her mental state), she may be suffering from the effects of one or more anticholinergic drugs.

"Natural" does not always mean "safe." Belladonna is derived from a plant known ominously as the *deadly nightshade.* Belladonna preparations—any anticholinergic medication for that matter—can be dangerous. Acute toxicity can make a person "dry as a bone, blind as a bat, red as a beet, and mad as a hatter." These symptoms result from belladonna's ability to

- block saliva production,
- interfere with sweating,
- paralyze eye muscles involved in near vision,
- increase blood flow to the skin, and
- create mental disturbance.

It's easy to attribute confusion, memory loss, or other decline in an older person's mental state to "old age" or dementia. The culprit may, in fact, be anticholinergic (or other) medication.

Keep in mind that an anticholinergic drug may be combined with others. For example, *orphenadrine* (Norflex) combined with aspirin and caffeine is sold as Norgesic.

Some people may be taking more than one anticholinergic drug at a given time, for example, diphenhydramine (Benadryl) for allergies and amitriptyline (Elavil) for pain, thereby increasing the likelihood of side effects.

Some Drugs With Anticholinergic Effects

Antivert .... *meclizine*
Artane .... *trihexyphenidyl*
Atarax .... *hydroxyzine*
Atrovent .... *ipratropium*
Benadryl .... *diphenhydramine*
Bentyl .... *dicyclomine*
Chlor-Trimeton ... *chlorpheniramine*
Cogentin .... *benztropine*
Compazine ...... *prochlorperazine*
Compoz .... *diphenhydramine*
Ditropan .... *oxybutynin*
Donnatal .... *belladonna + phenobarbital*
Dramamine ..... *dimenhydrinate*
Elavil .... *amitriptyline*
Flexeril .... *cyclobenzaprine*
Haldol .... *haloperidol*
Levsin .... *hyoscyamine*
Norflex .... *orphenadrine*
Nytol .... *diphenhydramine*
Periactin .... *cyproheptadine*
Phenergan ...... *promethazine*
Polaramine ...... *chlorpheniramine*
Pro-Banthine .... *propantheline*
Quinidex .... *quinidine*
Robinul .... *glycopyrrolate*
Sinequan .... *doxepin*
Spiriva .... *tiotropium*
Thorazine .... *chlorpromazine*
Vistaril .... *hydroxyzine*

Be on the alert. Anticholinergic drugs are everywhere. A partial list is included here. See Appendix C for a listing of anticholinergic drugs by therapeutic category.

Other Drugs, Other Effects

Sense of smell. A wide variety of medications are reported to reduce the sense of smell, which itself reduces the supply of saliva. These include *cholestyramine* (Questar), *cimetidine* (Tagamet), *gentamicin* (Gentacin), *levodopa* (Sinemet), *nifedipine* (Procardia), *phenylephrine* (Neo-Synephrine), *promethazine* (Phenergan), and *propythiouracil* (PTU).

Taste sensation. Drugs reported to interfere with the sense of taste include *alprazolam* (Xanax), *amitriptyline* (Elavil), *ampicillin*, *azathioprine* (Imuran), *baclofen* (Lioresal), *carbamazepine* (Tegretol), *colchicine*, *dilitiazem* (Cardizem), *doxepin* (Sinequan), *ethacrynic acid* (Edecrin), *hydrochlorothiazide* (Hydrodiuril), *hyoscyamine* (Levsin), *insulin*, *methotrexate*, *nitroglycerin*, *prednisone*, *propranolol* (Inderal), *spironolactone* (Aldactone), *sulfasalazine* (Azulfidine), and *vincristine*.

Level of alertness. Drugs used for agitation, allergies, anxiety, sleep, pain, and psychosis may cause drowsiness with resulting inattentiveness, impulsivity, and incoordination between breathing and swallowing.

Muscle movement. Several of the major tranquilizers—notably the phenothiazines *chlorpromazine* (Thorazine) and *thioridazine* (Mellaril)—have been associated with swallowing problems (including choking) linked with their effects upon muscle. They can, for example, cause too little movement (a Parkinson-like syndrome) or too much movement (tardive dyskinesia).

Microenvironment. Antibiotics used to treat pneumonia (and other infectious diseases) and drugs for cancer can alter the balance of microorganisms that normally live in the gastrointestinal tract, including the mouth. This can allow overgrowth of germs such as *candida*, causing a painful yeast infection of the mouth, called *thrush*.

Be Kind To Your Esophagus

The esophagus is exquisitely vulnerable to medication effects. Certain drugs can

- slow the movement of food and liquid through the esophagus
- irritate its lining to cause ulceration and scarring and
- keep the lower esophageal sphincter from closing, allowing acidic stomach contents to pass into the esophagus.

A pill that remains in the esophagus longer than the usual eight to twenty seconds will have a greater chance of injuring the *mucosa*, or lining. Damage to the esophageal mucosa can build up over months and years to cause a *stricture*, an encircling scar that interferes with passage of a bolus.

Chest discomfort or shoulder pain can signal esophageal injury. Keep in mind that these can be symptoms of a heart attack as well. So don't put off contacting your doctor or emergency medical services if the situation calls for it.

Drugs Known To Cause Esophageal Damage

alendronate	Fosamax
aspirin	ASA, acetylsalicylic acid
erythromycin	Ery Tab
ferrous sulfate (iron)	Feosol, Slow Fe
ibuprofen	Advil, Motrin
indomethacin	Indocin
potassium chloride	Kay Ciel, Slow-K
quinidine	Quinidex
theophylline	Theo-Dur
vitamin C	ascorbic acid

Some medications cause the lower esophageal sphincter to relax at the wrong time. Recall that the LES is contracted at rest. This prevents acidic stomach contents from flowing back into the esophagus where it can damage the mucosa and proceed from there to the throat.

81

Medications that promote relaxation of the lower esophageal sphincter include anticholinergic drugs, benzodiazepines, aminophylline, nitroglycerin, and beta-adrenergic agents such as *albuterol* (Proventil, Ventolin), *ipratropium* (Atrovent), and *terbutaline* (Brethine).

A Therapeutic Tightrope

The doctor often walks a fine line between therapeutic effects—such as relief of gastrointestinal distress, bronchial spasm, or muscular rigidity—and annoying or potentially dangerous side effects.

- *Dry mouth* can pave the way for a life-ending choking incident.
- *Blurry vision* can lead to a trip and fatal fall.
- *Rapid pulse* can cause cardiac decompensation and a heart attack.

Use your favorite search engine to check out side effects and interactions of prescribed and over-the-counter drugs. Be sure to discuss your findings and concerns with your doctor.

Making Pill-Taking Easier and Safer

The form of a medication may itself be a problem.

- Large pills (little "boulders") can get hung up traveling through the pharynx and esophagus.

- Gelatin capsules can stick to the throat or esophageal mucosa, especially when saliva is in short supply.
- Quick-dissolving medicines such as aspirin tablets without enteric coating can burn the esophagus.
- Small pills can hide out in pockets between cheek and gum or where a tooth is missing, ready to be aspirated.

Check with your swallowing specialist or pharmacist to see if you can replace a medication in tablet or capsule form with something better suited for your loved one.

Is the medication available as a liquid? In a smaller size or different shape? Can it be split, crushed, and sprinkled onto applesauce, pudding, or yogurt? A spoonful of applesauce can indeed help the medicine go down. For persons with diabetes or high blood pressure, be sure to keep an eye on the sugar and salt content of commercially prepared applesauce and pudding.

Once again, don't chop first and ask later. Some medicines, such as a long-acting form of *carbamazepine* (Tegretol), are designed to work *as a whole pill only*. Cut it in half and you destroy the drug-delivery system.

Take Special Care

Be sure to shake liquid medication vigorously prior to administration. The active part of the solution can settle to the bottom of the bottle after a few hours in the medicine cabinet.

If you don't shake the bottle well, the first doses will be diluted while the last will be concentrated. You'll be undertreating at the top of the bottle, overdosing at the bottom.

So, for liquid medication, the mantra is "Shake It, Shake It, Baby!"

Some medications bypass the oral route entirely. They are given as a suppository, by skin patch, by inhalation, or by injection.

A technique known as *effortful swallow* can help in taking pills (or for swallowing in general). This technique makes swallowing more consciously forceful. You are asked to concentrate, use your voluntary muscles, and "swallow hard"—like you're trying to swallow a golf ball.

Tips For Taking Medication

Here are some suggestions that can make pill-taking easier.

- Be calm.
- Breathe in a relaxed manner.
- Make sure your mouth is moist.
- Take one pill at a time.
- Place the pill toward the front of your tongue to reduce the tendency to gag.
- Take a good sip of water.
- Hold the pill and liquid in your mouth for a second or two.
- Tip chin to chest while swallowing
- Swallow consciously and forcefully.
- Relax between swallows and give yourself credit for a job well done.

It's *Not* Cool

It may look good on TV or in the movies, but you shouldn't throw your head back and toss pills to the back of your throat. They might wind up in your lungs.

If you need to tip your head back to get water from a cup or bottle, make sure you return to a level position before swallowing so you don't put yourself in a position to aspirate.

If you take pride in swallowing pills without water, be aware that this, too, is like playing with fire. It's a great way to set yourself up for choking or esophageal damage.

Always take pills with water or other liquid. Saliva is not enough. Once again, don't dry swallow pills!

Pill-Taking Anxiety

Fear can make taking medication an ordeal. The trauma of a childhood choking incident may extend into adulthood to cause difficulty swallowing pills.

Your uncle expects to have a problem getting his pills down. And sure enough, he does. In the blink of an eye he's anxious and aroused, ready for fight-or-flight. His mouth is dry, his throat tight.

Before concluding a swallowing problem is psychological, the doctor will rule out neurologic and structural causes of swallowing difficulty. Myasthenia gravis, for example, is notorious for being misdiagnosed as a purely psychological disorder.

When a swallowing problem is found to be emotionally-based, the speech-language pathologist will (1) work with the patient to increase knowledge and awareness of swallowing, (2) develop strategies that reduce the fear of swallowing, and (3) collaborate with a psychologist or psychiatrist.

A specially-designed cup can help a person swallow pills. With one particular cup, the pill sits in a chute that extends from the top of the cup to the person's mouth. When the cup is raised, the pill is carried by a comfortable gush of water through the lips to the back of the mouth, ready to be swallowed.

Your swallowing specialist will let you know if this or another specialized cup would be suitable for your loved one.

Water Matters

Some persons skimp on water when taking pills because they don't like to go to the bathroom frequently to urinate. It may be difficult or annoying for them to get there, or they may be incontinent.

Taking one pill at a time with a suitable amount of water can add up to significant fluid intake over the course of a day. That's something to keep in mind when a person has kidney disease or a heart condition and needs to keep a close eye on their fluids. A cup designed to deliver a pre-determined amount of fluid per sip (5 or 10 cc) may help in such circumstances.

Earlier If Possible

Try to schedule medication for as early in the day as possible, not right before bedtime. Lying down immediately after taking medication can lead to irritation of the esophagus and increase the risk of reflux.

While you're awake, up and about, you swallow saliva more often than when you're asleep. That helps move things through the esophagus. So, after taking medication, sit or, if permitted, walk for a few minutes.

Taking Medication Safely

Take the right pill at the right time.

Maintain hydration.

Watch for side effects of medication (such as dry mouth or drowsiness).

Don't toss or dry-swallow pills.

Shake liquid medication vigorously before each use.

Give medication by non-oral route, such as by skin patch, suppository, inhaler, or injection, as indicated.

Utilize the effortful swallow.

Use a specialized cup for swallowing pills, if permitted.

Watch for pills left behind after the swallow.

To address anxiety, work with a mental health professional as well as a swallowing specialist.

Take medication earlier in the day (not at bedtime) when possible.

Don't lie down immediately after taking medication.

In the next chapter, we will discuss treatment of swallowing problems.

CHAPTER 7

TREATING SWALLOWING PROBLEMS

TREATING SWALLOWING PROBLEMS

Treatment is not "one size fits all." It's individually tailored to meet the needs of your loved one. The swallowing specialist will look at the particulars of the swallowing problem and come up with a specific *treatment plan*.

The goals of treatment are

- to get to a state where swallowing is accomplished as safely as possible (minimizing the risk of choking or aspiration),
- to ensure adequate nutrition and hydration, and
- to accomplish the first two goals as pleasantly as possible.

Treatment does not take place in a vacuum. It involves the whole person as well as the family or other support system. Anything that improves a person's overall condition—strength, stamina, motivation, and emotional state—is likely to help with swallowing. And a safe, reliable swallow is likely to help overall condition.

The treatment plan begins with an *understanding* of what is wrong with swallowing. By this point, you should have a basic knowledge of swallowing, a sense of where things can go wrong, and why:

- a medical condition (congestive heart failure or pulmonary disease),
- a neurologic disorder (stroke or Parkinson disease),
- a structural problem (part of the tongue missing due to cancer surgery), and
- complicating effects of medication (dry mouth or altered sense of smell).

Whatever the swallowing issues may be, the *setting* is important. Close doors to reduce traffic (grandchildren, pets, repairmen, and the like).

If your loved one is easily distracted, turn off the TV and keep mealtime conversation to a minimum. It's perfectly fine, though, to provide reminders to chew thoroughly or carry out a particular swallowing maneuver. Don't forget to silence your cell phone.

We're not advocating an excessively somber atmosphere. But be careful about cracking jokes during a meal. Laughter (even talking) alters a person's breathing pattern and can cause an unsafe swallow.

Obviously, a person shouldn't eat (or be fed) if sleepy, confused, or agitated. Likewise, don't try to feed someone who is unusually weak or out of breath.

The Treatment Plan

- Understanding the problem
- The setting
- Positioning
- Proper food choices
- Safe swallowing strategies
- Diet modification
- Swallowing maneuvers
- Swallowing exercises
- Sensory stimulation
- Prostheses and surgery
- Oral care
- Pneumococcal vaccine
- Followup examination

Proper Positioning

Sitting upright, not tilted back or slumped to the side, helps breathing and swallowing. Sitting stably, feet on the floor if possible, facilitates breathing and feeding oneself.

If your mother takes her meals in bed, have her sit as upright as possible. Make sure her head does not fall back. Place pillows at her sides and behind her head so her trunk and head are straight.

Positioning *after* the meal is important, too. Don't rush your father to bed. A person should remain upright for thirty to forty-five minutes after eating or taking medication. This puts gravity to work, helping move the bolus through the esophagus and into the stomach, reducing the likelihood of aspiration and reflux.

Even if your loved one takes medication for reflux, don't count on that being 100 percent effective. At bedtime, elevate the upper part of the body 30 degrees by placing wedge pillows at the top of the bed to reduce the risk of reflux and aspiration during sleep.

Taking Care with Food and Drink

Avoid foods that have caused problems in the past, like steak, crusty bread, toast, popcorn, raw vegetables, whole nuts, banana, peanut butter, and pastries dusted with sugar.

Watch out for *foods of mixed consistency*. A mouthful of food may contain both liquid and solid elements. That can make swallowing tricky.

Consider dry cereal with milk. Your uncle may be able to handle cornflakes without a problem. But milk flowing willy-nilly to the back of his throat can cause him to cough and aspirate (see Fig. 7-1).

The solution may simply be to give the cornflakes time to get mushy. Less crunch, greater safety.

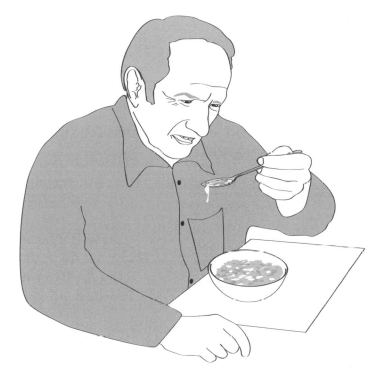

Figure 7-1: A Breakfast Challenge. Foods of mixed consistency—such as dry cereal with meal— can be dangerous.

What about salad? It certainly looks harmless. But salad can be hazardous. It can be difficult to reduce lettuce to a pasty, manageable bolus. Pieces stick to the tongue, hide out in the throat, or get trapped between cheek and gum in a position to be aspirated.

Salad dressing is an additional concern. As with milk and dry cereal, the vinaigrette can rush ahead of the lettuce to an unprotected airway and be sucked into the lungs with the next breath.

Likewise, be careful with fruit. They are usually of mixed consistency. Take a grape, for example. It's made up of skin, pulp, pit, and juice. All four must be reckoned with when it comes to chewing and swallowing.

Watch out, too, for carbonated beverages, which combine water and gas. Bubbles can tickle the throat to cause coughing or sneezing that interferes with the interplay between breathing and swallowing. The swallowing specialist may make soda a "No-no." Don't cheat.

Keep in mind that ice cream and some gelatin preparations start out as solids. But in a serving dish, in a spoon, or in the mouth, they melt to become a thin liquid—which your loved one may not be able to handle.

Mealtime Strategies

Involving the person you are caring for in the process of food preparation can get her psyched up for the meal. That helps build her appetite and promotes saliva flow, which we know is a good thing.

Take plenty of time for eating. A caregiver must realize that rushing through a meal is an invitation to aspiration or a choking disaster.

Eat a small amount at a time. Never has it been more true that you shouldn't bite off more than you can chew.

Chew thoroughly. We're not suggesting that you or your aunt count the number of chews. But we do recommend chewing until food reaches a soft, pasty, easy-to-swallow state.

Don't talk and eat at the same time. Talking is intimately connected with breathing. When you're excited about sharing something that's on your mind, it's easy to forget you have food or liquid in your mouth. So hold on to that thought and spare yourself a trip to the hospital.

Make sure that one swallow has been successfully completed before you begin another. After the swallow, make sure there's nothing left behind. Sweep the pockets between cheek and gum with the tongue (or finger, if necessary) to make sure nothing is left over that can be aspirated.

Alternate solids with liquids to moisten the mouth and throat. This helps move the bolus along and washes away food remnants.

Between swallows, clear the throat with a gentle cough, then swallow again. This helps remove food residue. Repeat as needed.

Arrange for smaller, more frequent meals if weakness, fatigue, or shortness of breath reduces the effectiveness of swallowing muscles. A person who eats with vigor at the start of a meal may become tired and distressed as the meal progresses.

Sip—Don't Guzzle or Gulp

As discussed in Chapter 3, drinking from a cup can be a challenge for many, especially for mouth-breathers. A series of gulps requires that breathing stop for several seconds, which can create considerable anxiety

Taking in a large amount of liquid at one time—gulping, guzzling, or chugging—can be risky for anyone with a swallowing problem. So, for the sake of safety as well as enjoyment, take it one sip at a time.

As mentioned in Chapter 6, specially designed cups can deliver a small, fixed amount of liquid per swallow.

Using a straw can help, too. But take care. A large squirt of liquid that arrives suddenly at the throat can cause a person to aspirate. Flexible straws allow for greater control. Be sure the straw is not too far back in the mouth and keep the sips small.

Therapeutic straws come in various sizes that require different pressures for sucking. Your swallowing specialist will let you know whether such straws are appropriate—or whether any straw is advisable.

Be On the Lookout

At all times, watch for signs of distress (such as choking, coughing, tearing, or regurgitation through the nose). Be ready to carry out the Heimlich maneuver if necessary (see Chapter 4).

Watch the Adam's apple. Does it go all the way up with the swallow? If it doesn't, be suspicious that the swallow was ineffective. Food may still be in the throat.

Have the person swallow again. If the Adam's apple does move, that's a good sign—though it takes a swallowing specialist to know if it moves *enough*.

Don't reload the fork or spoon until you're confident that a successful swallow has been completed. Remember—no food should be left behind.

Diet Modification

Modification of the diet can be a cornerstone of the treatment plan. It is, however, something that many people fear. But if you understand why it is being called into play, you can explain to your loved one and others involved in providing care why it is necessary at this time.

Let's say, for example, your aunt has been found to aspirate "thin" liquids such as juice or tea and this has led to two episodes of pneumonia. Mixing these drinks with a taste-free thickening agent will allow her greater control in swallowing and can reduce the risk of aspiration.

Liquids are categorized as thin (like water), nectar-thick, honey-thick, and pudding-thick. Thickening agents or prepared drinks are readily available through your local pharmacy or online providers.

Changing the consistency of solid foods, too, can make swallowing safer. Softer foods place fewer demands upon jaw muscles that are weak or tire easily. Ground meat, tofu, and pudding don't require much of loosely fitting dentures. Plus, these foods are kinder to inflamed cheek and gum tissues.

It Can Get Emotional

People don't like to hear about changes in their diet. They often feel that something precious is being taken away from them.

We understand. At this point, they may have lost many of their most private and personal habits, routines, and pleasures. When a change in diet is recommended, they often respond emotionally—with fear, anger, or denial.

The thought of "baby food" three times a day can bring a person to despair. "All purée all the time" is not a pleasant prospect.

For now, however, the change may be necessary for their survival—to prevent choking and aspiration while ensuring nutrition and hydration. The dietary change may not be permanent. That will depend upon the particular swallowing problem and the response to treatment.

For those who require a modified diet, they should know there's a lot of delicious food available. See the **Notes** for this chapter for two excellent cookbooks.

Swallowing Maneuvers

As directed by your swallowing specialist, maneuvers of the head and neck can facilitate swallowing. A common maneuver is the *chin tuck*, also called the *chin-down posture*. This involves tucking the chin to the chest while swallowing. The therapist may assist with a gentle touch to the head.

Keep in mind that maintaining eye contact with a caregiver can interfere with the chin tuck maneuver. So if you are feeding your mother, you may want to bow your head and break eye contact momentarily to avoid this problem.

Another maneuver involves turning the head to one side during the swallow. With stroke patients this maneuver takes advantage of swallowing muscles that continue to function relatively normally, working around the paralyzed side and exploiting gravity. The therapist may combine these maneuvers with an *effortful swallow* (see Chapter 6).

Exercises for Swallowing

Muscles of the face, tongue, lips, cheeks, and larynx can be exercised to enhance speed, range of motion, strength, and endurance. Involving muscles of the abdomen and chest helps, too, because of their role in breathing and coughing.

Even the upper esophageal sphincter can benefit from exercise. Lying flat and elevating the head according to the Shaker ("shah-KAIR") exercise protocol can extend the time that the upper esophageal sphincter stays open, allowing for a safer, more complete passage of a bolus.

Regular visits to the "swallowing gym" can be supplemented by "dance lessons" devoted to improving coordination of muscles involved in swallowing and breathing.

Even though they're not running a mile, elderly persons with cardiac and respiratory conditions should take special care when it comes to swallowing exercises. Such exercises may simply be too strenuous. Check with your doctor and swallowing specialist before embarking upon any exercise program.

Keep in mind that participating in an exercise program requires understanding, attention, and motivation. Persons with cognitive limitations, such as those associated with advanced Alzheimer disease or following severe head trauma, will generally require cognitive as well as swallowing therapy.

Once the speech-language pathologist has developed a suitable exercise program, she can instruct family members and other caregivers in carrying out this part of the treatment plan.

Sensory Stimulation

The swallowing reflex—indeed, *any* reflex—depends upon sensation. If the throat cannot detect the presence of food, the swallowing reflex will not be triggered. Food can remain dangerously behind, putting a person at risk of choking or aspiration.

To enhance the sensory arm of the swallowing reflex, the therapist may use an ice-cold cotton-tipped applicator dipped in lemon juice to stimulate the throat. This technique of *thermal-tactile stimulation* can make the swallow brisker and stronger not just once but several times after a single application.

Stimulation of the throat by means of electrodes applied to the skin (*transcutaneous electrical stimulation*) appears to benefit some persons with swallowing difficulty.

"Nothing By Mouth"

Under some circumstances, it may be necessary to bypass swallowing altogether for a period of time. After a stroke, for example, a person may be required to take "nothing by mouth"—or, in medical lingo, to be "NPO," from the Latin *nil per os.*

For shorter-term use, say, thirty days or less, a *nasogastric tube* extending from nose to stomach may be used for feeding.

For longer periods, a tube may be placed directly into the stomach. This is called a *gastrostomy tube,* or *G-tube*. Because it is inserted by way of an endoscope, it is commonly known as a *PEG-tube*, for *percutaneous endoscopic gastrostomy*.

Keep in mind that even with tube feeding a person can aspirate. The combination of saliva, bacteria, and a faulty swallowing mechanism can result in aspiration pneumonia.

Diet modification and tube feeding can serve as a *bridge to the future*—a future with a functional, relatively safe swallow. Many stroke patients, for example, will be able to resume eating a normal diet within a few weeks to a few months. So be patient. Follow the treatment plan.

While healing and therapy are underway, your understanding and support as a loving caregiver can help prevent dangerous slip-ups. Make sure your family knows, as you do, why sneaking a cheeseburger to Uncle Billy for his birthday—while he's recovering from a stroke—will not be doing him a favor. It could cost him his life.

Prostheses and Surgery

In some patients with head and neck cancer, a prosthetic soft palate can be designed to prevent nasal regurgitation. For palatal paralysis after a stroke, surgical attachment of the paralyzed portion to the throat can reduce nasal regurgitation and lessen the risk of aspiration.

Direct injection of botulinum toxin into the lower esophageal sphincter can cause it to relax, allowing for months of symptomatic benefit. Surgical procedures include stretching or cutting the LES to widen it.

Depending upon a person's symptoms, a Zenker diverticulum may require surgical treatment.

Oral Care Counts!

The mouth, gums, and dentures provide a fertile environment for germs that can make their way from mouth to lungs to cause life-threatening aspiration pneumonia.

That's why a regular program of in-house oral care—at least two times per day—is so important. Oral care includes the use of a toothbrush (manual or electric) for teeth and dentures; swabs to moisturize and soothe the lips, tongue, and cheeks; mouth rinses containing antibacterial agents (as directed by the dentist); and suctioning of pooled saliva, which is likely to be teeming with bacteria.

The oral care program should be combined with regular dental visits and professional cleanings.

Another thing you can do to help prevent pneumonia that results from aspiration of oral and pharyngeal contents is to discuss the use of pneumococcal vaccine with your loved one's primary physician.

Suggestions for Safe Swallowing

We've put together a set of wide-ranging suggestions that can help your loved one swallow more safely (see Appendix B). They touch upon the following:

- the mental and physical state of the person you're caring for
- the setting
- positioning
- food preparation
- mealtime strategies
- taking medication comfortably and safely
- things to do after meals
- things to do between meals.

Not all suggestions will apply to every situation. Highlight those you consider most useful, or transfer to another sheet of paper. Check with your swallowing specialist as to what suits your particular circumstances.

Post your list in the kitchen, dining room, or other eating area. Copy and share with other caregivers.

Ongoing Evaluation and Treatment

Treatment of swallowing problems is an ongoing process. Several sessions over several months may be required to meet treatment goals.

The initial plan may not be the final plan. The swallowing specialist will follow the patient over time, monitoring progress at the bedside or in the office. She will arrange for further testing as needed and make necessary adjustments to the diet.

Be sure to keep the doctor, nurse, and swallowing specialist informed as to advance directives and changes in your loved one's condition. If you think the treatment plan is no longer suitable, let them know your concerns as soon as possible.

In the next chapter, we show you how to put your questions, observations, and concerns to use in getting help for your loved one.

CHAPTER 8

GETTING HELP

GETTING HELP

A t this point, you probably have a sense as to whether your mother or your father—or you—have a swallowing problem. Perhaps an evaluation has been carried out and treatment begun. If not, it's time to take action.

In this chapter, we show you how to gather your concerns and observations to get the help your loved one needs. We've set up a *Letter For Your Doctor* you can use to record key information (see Appendix A).

You can indicate, for example, how long you've observed such symptoms as difficulty swallowing, voice change after eating, and frequent throat-clearing. You can list overall medical problems, recent hospitalizations, and current medications.

Fill it out with your spouse, another family member, a friend, a professional caregiver, or by yourself. Make a copy of this letter for yourself. Bring it to the next doctor's visit. Or mail, fax, or hand-deliver it in advance to the primary medical provider (internist, geriatrician, family physician, general practitioner, nurse practitioner, or physician's assistant).

Ask when you can expect a reply. Write that date down as a reminder to call if you haven't heard by then.

Your letter may prompt the doctor to have you bring your mother to the office as a first step. Or he may refer her straight away to a swallowing specialist without seeing her.

If things worsen at any time—if she has greater difficulty swallowing, threatened dehydration, labored breathing, or progressive weakness, for example—seek prompt medical attention.

The Swallowing Specialist

The doctor may refer your mother to a *speech-language pathologist*. "But there's nothing wrong with my speech!" she protests.

That may or may not be true. It turns out that many of the same structures we use for speaking are also used for swallowing—all of which fall within the realm of speech-language pathology. The specialist will probably have the initials CCC-SLP after her name. They stand for Certificate of Clinical Competence in Speech-Language Pathology.

This certification means that she (or he) has successfully completed a rigorous training program (usually two to three years, at a master's or Ph.D. level) followed by an additional year of supervised clinical fellowship. The specialist has also passed a national qualifying examination with certification through the American Speech-Language-Hearing Association (ASHA).

Speech-language pathologists work in a variety of settings. These include hospitals, nursing homes, assisted living facilities, patients' homes, or private offices. Some speech-language pathologists have made swallowing an area of special expertise.

Examination of Swallowing

The initial swallowing evaluation will probably be carried out in an office or at the bedside. Through conversation, the speech-language pathologist (SLP) gathers information not just about swallowing but about the *whole* person: educational background, occupation (past or present), interests, family structure, and support system.

These are some of the questions the SLP addresses:

- Is the patient alert or drowsy?
- Oriented to person, place, and time?
- Calm or anxious?
- Focused, or easily distracted?
- How is memory for recent and past events?
- Is hearing adequate for conversation?
- Does she breathe comfortably through her nose or effortfully through the mouth?
- Is breathing shallow, rapid, or irregular?

- Is there a dry or rattling cough? Wheezing?
- How is the posture? Hunched at the shoulders or tilted to one side?
- Is there a tremor of the hands or voice?
- Is the person malnourished or obese?
- Do sticky lips and a dry tongue suggest dehydration?
- How are strength, balance, coordination, and mobility of the head, shoulders, neck, arms, and hands?
- Is the voice strong and full, or weak?
- Is it nasal?
- Is speech fluent and intelligible?
- Does the patient understand the questions that are asked?
- Does he understand his personal medical condition?
- Is he aware of swallowing difficulty?
- Does the patient appear able to follow a treatment plan?
- Is a caregiver available to provide assistance?

The swallowing specialist will inspect oral structures. Are teeth missing? Are dentures securely in place? Is the tongue moist? Is the inside of cheeks a healthy pink or marred by white patches?

This inspection is followed by an *oral motor examination*, which focuses on muscles involved in swallowing: the face, lips, tongue, jaw, soft palate, throat, and larynx.

Next comes an examination of swallowing itself. If the examiner considers it safe, she will offer small amounts of food and liquid of different consistencies to see how the patient handles them.

These are some of the things the examiner watches for:

- Is the swallow forceful?
- Does the Adam's apple rise with the swallow?
- Does the person need more than one swallow to get the food down?
- Does food remain on the tongue or in the throat after the swallow?
- Does the patient cough before, during, or after the swallow?
- Does the voice change afterwards?
- Does the nose run after swallowing?
- Does the patient feel that food gets stuck? If so, where?
- How is the coordination between breathing and chewing? Between breathing and swallowing?
- Does the patient have difficulty with liquids, solids, or both?

A bedside or office examination of swallowing may include measurement of oxygen saturation. This is accomplished painlessly by means of a sensor placed around a finger. A decrease in oxygen saturation suggests that food or liquid is getting into the respiratory system, supporting the likelihood of aspiration.

Immediate Treatment and Further Testing

The swallowing specialist may put protective measures into place at once to reduce the risk of choking and aspiration. These measures might include diet modification and swallowing maneuvers discussed in the previous chapter. She may also recommend further testing such as a chest x-ray or a specialized test of swallowing.

A chest x-ray by itself does not directly identify a swallowing problem, though a particular pattern of pneumonia on an x-ray can suggest aspiration as the cause. Be aware that a chest x-ray may not show pneumonia soon after a person has aspirated. So, if the chest x-ray is normal, don't assume that aspiration has been ruled out or that all is well with swallowing.

Specialized Tests of Swallowing

More specific diagnostic tests may be called upon to (1) confirm the clinical suspicion of aspiration, (2) clarify at what phase of swallowing it occurs,

(3) determine what foods and liquids the patient handles best, and (4) identify postures and maneuvers that facilitate safe swallowing.

Two of the tests used to visualize swallowing are the *modified barium swallow* and *fiberoptic endoscopic evaluation of swallowing*.

The *barium swallow*, also known as an *upper GI series*, looks primarily at the upper digestive tract in investigating such problems as ulcer and cancer. It can help diagnose some swallowing problems, but does not look at all phases of swallowing.

The *modified barium swallow* (MBS), on the other hand, *does* look at all phases of swallowing, from preparatory through esophageal. The patient swallows small amounts of food and liquid—a cookie or applesauce, for example—mixed with barium. Since barium shows up clearly on x-ray film, the entire swallow can be recorded digitally or on videotape.

The modified barium swallow, or *videofluoroscopic swallowing study*, is typically conducted by a radiologist and a speech-language pathologist. It looks at how a person handles food and liquids of different consistency and generally includes maneuvers such as changes in head position during the swallow to see if these will benefit the patient. The MBS usually takes thirty minutes to an hour to complete.

Fiberoptic endoscopic evaluation of swallowing (FEES) does not involve x-rays. A specialist passes a thin endoscope—a tube containing a tiny camera—through the nose to allow for direct visualization of parts of the swallow, primarily its pharyngeal stage. FEES also permits assessment of sensation of key structures involved in swallowing.

Overview of the Clinical Process

Obtain history of swallowing problem

Elicit present and past medical, neurologic, and psychiatric history

Bedside or office examination of swallowing

Investigation by means of chest x-ray, MBS, or FEES

Treatment that might include diet modification, positioning, swallowing maneuvers, exercises, prosthesis, or surgery

Further specialist evaluation

Follow-up examination

Modification of treatment plan as needed

The Swallowing Team

In addition to a speech-language pathologist, other specialists often take part in evaluating and treating a person with swallowing problems. They might include one (or more) of the following: an ear-nose-

and-throat specialist, neurologist, oncologist, dentist, gastroenterologist, or rheumatologist.

Other health professionals who might be engaged include a physical therapist (who works on body posture, balance, strength, and breathing) and an occupational therapist (to guide patients and caregivers in the mechanics of eating). A nutritionist and pharmacist often collaborate as well.

Difficult Decisions

Some of you reading this book will be grappling with complicated, often wrenching, quality-of-life and end-of-life issues pertaining to a loved one. Because swallowing is so closely related to nutrition and to dangers of choking, aspiration, and pneumonia, it often becomes a focus of decision-making. Issues may relate to tube-feeding, intravenous hydration, and diet modification.

After a swallowing problem has been identified and a treatment plan developed, the patient (or suitably-designated decision-maker) may wish to pursue a course of action that differs from that recommended by the specialist.

Take for example a woman who, after several bouts of pneumonia, was found to aspirate thin liquids. Aspiration was diagnosed on the basis of bedside examination confirmed by a modified barium swallow. Thickened liquids were recommended to lessen the risk of aspiration.

119

She tried to drink her beloved coffee, now thickened, but couldn't stand the texture. "I'm not drinking that!" she let it be known. She understood that she had a swallowing problem and a tendency to aspirate; to continue drinking coffee as she preferred could lead to further pneumonia or worse.

She discussed the matter with her family and swallowing specialist. To make things as clear as possible, she put her thoughts, feelings, desires, and intentions in writing.

Understanding the risks, she chose to continue to drink her coffee "undoctored"—without any thickener. She would do so in as safe a manner as possible. For her, that meant sipping slowly, tucking chin to chest while swallowing, clearing her throat after the swallow, and swallowing again before taking another sip.

A patient who rejects the recommendation of a specialist or the swallowing team can present a dilemma for physicians, nurses, and therapists committed to ethical principles of their professions while respecting the position of the patient and family.

In situations such as these it may be valuable to consult with an elder care lawyer, social worker, psychologist, psychiatrist, priest, minister, rabbi, or other clergyperson to help clarify matters.

An Advance Directive

The individual and family may choose a health care proxy to make health care decisions on behalf of that individual should he or she become incapacitated. An advance medical directive might specify, for example, that modification of liquids and solid foods would be allowed, but not tube feeding of any kind.

Seeing to it that the wishes of your loved one are dealt with in a manner most appropriate for him or her can reduce everybody's anxiety and allow your loved one to lead the fullest life possible.

Your Crucial Role as Caregiver

Throughout the diagnostic and therapeutic process, keep in mind the unique and vital role you play—as spouse, child, or friend.

What you observe at home or at a care center provides the physician and swallowing specialist with important information they are not able to gain directly, information that helps them manage these complex situations.

It is your love that guides you to learn more, your caring that ensures that recommendations are carried out as fully as possible, your patience and strength that enable you to be with someone you love through difficult times.

You help establish and maintain a safe environment for your loved one.

You help him or her understand what the problems are and what to do about them.

You help to prepare nutritious and tasty foods that are best suited to their needs.

You help your loved one use safe swallowing strategies.

You help them practice their exercises.

You help them take their pills comfortably and safely.

You help them reduce the risk of choking, aspiration, pneumonia, and malnutrition.

You are the glue that holds it all together.

CHAPTER 9

MINDFUL
SWALLOWING

MINDFUL
SWALLOWING

We hope that by now you've developed a feel for swallowing problems and what to do about them.

Keep learning. Don't stop observing or asking questions. Be prepared at all times for a choking emergency. If and when you do encounter a problem or have a concern, we trust that you know what to do.

We realize there's no absolute way to protect everyone from every swallowing problem. We feel, though, that knowing how swallowing works and how things can go wrong, you're in a good position to recognize, deal with, and prevent swallowing problems that can affect an elderly person, younger adults with medical or neurologic disorders, your children, or yourself.

Attention, Boomers!

Many of you reading this book are Baby Boomers—between the ages of about 45 and 65—participating in the care of an elderly parent, a spouse, or an adult child. Share this book with them and with others involved in their care.

You can do a few simple things to help your loved ones stay out of harm's way. Remind them about the importance of not rushing through meals, eating food in small bites, chewing well, finishing a swallow before speaking, and other things you've learned in this book.

If you suspect a swallowing problem, don't delay in arranging for evaluation. The next incident might be a fatal choking episode or aspiration leading to pneumonia that puts your mother or father into the hospital, never to return home.

Contact the primary medical provider as soon as possible. Use the *Letter For Your Doctor* to record your observations and concerns.

Day To Day With Your Family

As you sit down at mealtime with your family, take pleasure in the setting and the company. Enhance your relationship with your spouse. Develop a stronger bond with your children.

Eating breakfast and listening to the radio while checking your e-mail is all too common these days. Nothing gets your full attention. Little good can come from that. Save your multitasking for later.

If you are mindful while eating—engaged in the present—you will likely enjoy your food more, chew it better, and eat less than if you are mindlessly shoveling it in.

When it comes to celebrating at home or in a restaurant, be aware that risks can be multiplied. Talking, laughing, drinking alcohol, and swallowing make for a dangerous combination.

So slow down. Take a breath. Relax. Smell your food. Taste it. Chew thoroughly. Feel the food change from solid to soft. Enjoy the process, and....**SWALLOW SAFELY!**

Appendix A

Letter
For Your Doctor

Appendix A: Letter For Your Doctor

Date_____

Dear Doctor_____

I am concerned about swallowing in

_____   _____

Name of Person   Date of Birth

She/He is my: mother   father   wife   husband

other _____

I have noticed these problems over the past

_____ weeks/months. (Circle those that apply)

difficulty swallowing   coughing   choking   gagging

wheezing   tearing of eyes   runny nose   chest pain

nasal regurgitation   weight loss   fever   sore throat

voice change: hoarse   weak   gargly   nasal

frequent throat-clearing   tired out by eating   nausea

food feels stuck/won't go down   drooling   heartburn

eating very slowly   dehydration   refusing food

loose dentures   sore gums   bad breath

other _____

From SWALLOW SAFELY www.swallowsafely.com

SWALLOW SAFELY

She/He has these medical problems:

_____

_____

_____

Her/His last hospitalization was _____ (date)

at _____(hospital)

for these reasons:_____

_____

She/He is taking the following medications

(prescribed and over-the-counter):

_____

_____

_____

I am most concerned about: choking   aspiration

pneumonia   nutrition   hydration

difficulty swallowing pills

Other_____

_____

Appendix A: Letter For Your Doctor

I look forward to hearing from you at your earliest convenience.

You can reach me in the following ways:

Home Phone   (   )_____

Cell phone   (   )_____

Fax   (   )_____

E-mail _____

Mailing Address _____

_____

Thank you very much for your attention and concern.

       Sincerely,

           _____
                     Your signature

          _____
                   Your name printed

APPENDIX B

———◆·◆———

SUGGESTIONS
FOR SAFE SWALLOWING

SUGGESTIONS
FOR SAFE SWALLOWING

MENTAL AND PHYSICAL STATE

- Don't eat if drowsy, confused, or agitated.
- Don't eat if unusually weak or out of breath.

SETTING

- Reduce distractions: Turn off TV, radio, cell phone.
- Relaxing music is OK.
- Close doors to reduce traffic.
- Don't overdo conversation or promote laughter while eating.

POSITIONING

- Sit upright, not tilted back or slumped to the side.
- Provide firm support for legs.

FOOD PREPARATION

- Involve the person with a swallowing problem in preparing food to promote saliva flow and overall enthusiasm for eating.
- Check temperature of food and liquids to make sure they are not excessively hot or annoyingly cold.
- Avoid difficult-to-swallow foods such as crusty bread, toast, popcorn, raw vegetables (celery, lettuce, etc.), whole nuts, and peanut butter.

- Avoid crumbly, flaky foods and pastries dusted with sugar.
- Be careful with (or avoid altogether) carbonated beverages.
- Watch out for foods of mixed consistency such as some fruit and cereal with milk.
- Be careful with foods (like ice cream or Jello) that melt.
- Avoid foods or liquids that have caused prior difficulty.
- Provide tasty foods of suitable consistency.
- Thicken liquids as directed.

MEALTIME STRATEGIES

- Don't rush.
- Eat a small amount at a time.
- Chew thoroughly.
- Don't talk and eat at the same time.
- Use the chin tuck maneuver, as directed.
- Swallow, clear throat with a gentle cough, and swallow again before taking in more food.
- Finish the swallow before reloading spoon or fork.
- After the swallow, check mouth for left-over food or pill.
- Clear the mouth, if needed, by tongue, hand, or mechanical suction.
- Alternate solids and liquids to facilitate passage of the bolus and wash away residue.
- Watch for fatigue; finish meal another time, if necessary.
- Arrange for smaller, more frequent meals.
- Note cough, sputter, choke, gag, tearing, runny nose, nasal regurgitation, or other problems.
- If someone coughs or chokes, do not slap on the back.
- Be prepared to carry out the Heimlich maneuver.

- If a choking person leaves the room, *follow him or her.* Do not leave alone until the incident is resolved.

TAKING MEDICATION

- Stay calm.
- Sit upright.
- Take one pill at a time.
- Swallow pills with plenty of liquid to make swallowing easier and to protect the esophagus.
- Don't exceed daily fluid requirements.
- Use applesauce to facilitate pill-taking.
- Replace difficult-to-swallow pills with more suitable preparations, as approved by a pharmacist.
- Use a specialized cup, if allowed.
- Take medications as early in the day as possible.
- Remain upright for 30 minutes after taking pills.
- In general, use the same strategies that work for swallowing solids and liquids (e.g., effortful swallow, chin tuck).

AFTER MEALS

- Do not lie down for 30-45 minutes after eating.
- Walk for several minutes if permitted.
- Clean teeth, gums, and dentures several times per day.
- Use an antibacterial mouth rinse as prescribed.
- Swab lips, tongue, and cheeks to moisturize and lubricate the mouth.
- Suction pooled saliva to reduce the bacterial load.
- Arrange for regular dental care.

BETWEEN MEALS

- Watch for respiratory difficulty (such as cough, rapid breathing, or wheezing), chest pain, or voice change.

139

SWALLOW SAFELY

- Carry out approved swallowing-related exercises that involve breathing, coughing, and chewing.
- Work on overall fitness, muscle strength, balance, and posture.
- Keep mind and body active with reading, playing bridge and Scrabble, doing word puzzles and Sudoku, mentoring, and other activities.
- At bedtime, elevate the head of bed to 30 degrees to help prevent aspiration or reflux during sleep.

APPENDIX C

ANTICHOLINERGIC DRUGS BY CATEGORY

ANTICHOLINERGIC DRUGS
BY CATEGORY

Antihistamines
chlorpheniramine	Chlor-Trimeton, Polaramine
cyproheptadine	Periactin
dimenhydrinate	Dramamine
diphenhydramine	Benadryl, Compoz, Nytol, Unisom
hydroxyzine	Atarax, Vistaril
promethazine	Phenergan

Antiparkinsonian
benztropine	Cogentin
procyclidine	Kemadrin
trihexyphenidyl	Artane

Antivertigo
meclizine	Antivert
prochlorperazine	Compazine
promethazine	Phenergan

Cardiac
disopyramide	Norpace
procainamide	Procanbid
quinidine	Cardioquin, Quinidex, Quinora

143

Gastrointestinal

belladonna preparations (containing atropine, hyoscine, hyoscyamine, or scopolamine)

	Donnatal (includes phenobarbital)
glycopyrrolate	Robinul
hyoscyamine	Levsin
propantheline	Pro-Banthine
dicyclomine	Bentyl

Herbal Preparations

Atropa belladonna (deadly nightshade)
Brugmansia species (Angel's trumpet)
Datura stramonium (datura)
Hyoscyamus niger (henbane)
Mandragora officinarum (mandrake)

Pain Relievers

cylcobenzaprine	Flexeril
methocarbamol	Robaxin
orphenadrine	Norflex

Psychiatric

Major Tranquilizers/Antipsychotics

chlorpromazine	Thorazine
clozapine	Clozaril
fluphenazine	Prolixin
haloperidol	Haldol
perphenazine	Trilafon
thioridazine	Mellaril
thiothixene	Navane

Appendix C: Anticholinergic Drugs By Category

Antidepressants

amitriptyline	Elavil
clomipramine	Anafranil
desipramine	Norpramine
imipramine	Tofranil
nortriptyline	Aventyl, Pamelor
doxepin	Sinequan

Respiratory

ipratropium	Atrovent
tiotropium	Spiriva

Urinary Tract

oxybutynin	Ditropan
tolterodine	Detrol

APPENDIX D

———◆———

WHAT'S YOUR
SWALLOWING STORY?

If you have a swallowing story you'd like to share with us (confidentially, of course) or would like to ask us a question, you can reach us by e-mail at swallowsafely@aol.com or by mail:

Roya Sayadi and Joel Herskowitz
Inside/Outside Press
P.O. Box 661
Natick, MA 01760

We look forward to hearing from you.

NOTES

Chapter 1. Why We Wrote This Book

3. *Many people....falling in the elderly:* Tinetti ME: Preventing falls in elderly persons. *New England Journal of Medicine* (2003) 348:42-49.

Tinetti ME, Kumar C: The patient who falls: "It's always a trade-off." *Journal of the American Medical Association* (2010) 303:258-266.

3. *Account for nearly:* Centers for Disease Control and Prevention (CDC): Falls among older adults: An overview. Updated Oct. 6, 2009. http://www.cdc.gov/HomeandRecreationalSafety/falls/adultfalls.html

3. *You do many things:* National Institute on Aging (NIA): Falls and fractures. Updated Nov. 4, 2009. http://www.nia.nih.gov/Health Information/Publications/falls.htm

Perkins-Carpenter B: *How To Prevent Falls: Better Balance, Independence and Energy in 6 Simple Steps.* Senior Fitness Productions, Inc., Penfield, NY, 2006.

3. *Account for tens of thousands of deaths:* Murry T, Carrau RL, Eibling DE: "Epidemiology of Swallowing Disorders," Chapter 1, in *Comprehensive Management of Swallowing Disorders,* Carrau RL, Murry T (eds.), Singular Publishing Group, Inc., San Diego, CA, 1999, pp. 3-7.

Robbins JA, Gensler G, Hind J, Logemann JA, Lindblad AS, Brandt D, Baum H, Lilienfeld D, Kosek S, Lundy D, Dikeman K, Kazandjian M, Gramigna GD, McGarvey-Toler S, Miller Gardner PJ: Comparison of 2 interventions for liquid aspiration on pneumonia incidence: A randomized trial. *Annals of Internal Medicine* (2008) 148:509-18. http://www.annals.org/content/148/7/509.full.pdf+html?sid=a67b0803-8f8e-45d3-b2b1-a62cc2f00867

4. *Choking takes....lives:* Warshawsky ME: Foreign body aspiration. *emedicine.* Updated Jan. 3, 2008. http://emedicine.medscape.com/article/298940-overview

4. *Aspiration of food, liquid:* Marik PE, Kaplan D: Aspiration pneumonia and dysphagia in the elderly. *Chest* (2003) 124:328-36. http://chestjournal.chestpubs.org/content/124/1/328.abstract?ijkey=3f c1c4e333fcf244880f14928f4ec9b297eb4e6a&keytype2=tf_ipsecsha

Medina-Walpole AM, Katz PR: Nursing home-acquired pneumonia. *Journal of the American Geriatrics Society* (1999) 47:1005-15.

Murry T, Carrau RL: "The Abnormal Swallow: Conditions and Diseases." Part III, in *Clinical Management of Swallowing Disorders, Second Edition.* Plural Publishing, Inc., San Diego, CA, 2006, p, 47.

4. *Malnutrition resulting from:* Evans, C: Malnutrition in the elderly: A multifactorial failure to thrive. *Permanente Journal* (2005) 9:38-41. *http:/xnet.kp.org/permanentejournal/sum05/elderly.pdf*

4. *Nearly 40 million Americans:* U.S. Census Bureau: The Older Population in the United States: 2008. http://www.census.gov/ population/www/socdemo/age/older_2008.html

4. *And older. From 15 to 50 percent:* Robbins J: The current state of clinical geriatric dysphagia research. *Journal of Rehabilitation Research & Development* (2002) 39:vii-ix. http://www.rehab. research.va.gov/jour/02/39/4/pdf/guested.pdf

4. *Somewhere between....and growing:* Hobbs FB: The elderly population. In "Population Profile of the United States." U.S. Census Bureau, last modified July 8, 2008. *http:/www.census.gov/ population/www/pop-profile/elderpop.html*

4. *Swallowing problems....billions of dollars:* Boyce JM, Potter-Bynoe G, Dziobek L, RN; Solomon SL: Nosocomial pneumonia in Medicare patients: Hospital costs and reimbursement patterns under the prospective payment system. *Archives of Internal Medicine* (1991) 151:1109-14.

Katzan IL, Dawson NV, Thomas CL, Votruba ME, Cebul RD: The cost of pneumonia after acute stroke. *Neurology* (2007) 68:1938-43. http://www.neurology.org/cgi/content/abstract/68/22/1938

6. *Typical Scenarios:* These examples are composites of clinical situations. Hence any link with a particular person would be coincidental.

Notes

7. *A typical patient:* Carpenter S: Treating an illness is one thing. What about a patient with many? *The New York Times*, March 31, 2009. http://www.nytimes.com/2009/03/31/health/31sick.html

7. *Would be for....a dozen medications:* Gorard DA: Escalating polypharmacy. *Quarterly Journal of Medicine* (2006) 99:797-800. http://qjmed.oxfordjournals.org/cgi/reprint/99/11/797

9. *Because swallowing is vital:* Sharp HM, Bryant KN: Ethical issues in dysphagia: When patients refuse assessment or treatment. *Seminars in Speech and Language* (2003) 24:285-99.

10. *Having cared for:* Winakur J: What are we going to do with Dad? A geriatrician stands by during his father's downward spiral into old age, disability, and dementia. *Health Affairs* (2005) 24:1064-1072. http://content.healthaffairs.org/cgi/content/full/24/4/1064

10. *Swallowing problems:* Greenberg J: Dangerous disorders of swallowing are common but subtle. *New York Times*, Sept. 1, 1981. http://www.nytimes.com/1981/09/01/science/dangerous-disorders-of-swallowing-are-common-but-subtle.html

Chapter 2. How Swallowing Works

15. *And-gone. It's a process:* Aviv JE: "The Normal Swallow," Chapter 3, in *Comprehensive Management of Swallowing Disorders*, Carrau RL, Murry T (eds.), Singular Publishing Group, Inc., San Diego, CA, 1999, pp. 23-29.

Linkinhoker M: Swallowing, An Animated Sequence. Johns Hopkins Gastroenterology and Hepatology Resource Center, Johns Hopkins University; Link Studio, LLC, Baltimore, MD. http://www.linkstudio.info/portfolio/interact07c1.htm

Logemann JA: "Anatomy and Physiology of Normal Deglutition." Chapter 2, in *Evaluation and Treatment of Swallowing Disorders*, *2nd edition*, PRO-ED, Inc., Austin, TX, 1998, pp. 13-35.

17. *Likewise, breathing and swallowing:* Martin-Harris B, Brodsky MB, Michel Y, Ford CL, Walters B, Heffner J: Breathing and swallowing dynamics across the adult lifespan. *Archives of Otolaryngology—Head and Neck Surgery* (2005) 131:762-70. http://archotol.ama-assn.org/cgi/content/full/131/9/762

22. *A word....about gagging:* Ramsey DJC, Smithard DG, Kalra L: Early Assessments of Dysphagia and Aspiration Risk in Acute Stroke Patients. *Stroke* (2003) 34:1252-57. http://stroke.ahajournals. org/cgi/reprint/34/5/1252

Chapter 3. When Swallowing Doesn't Work

29. *Before going any further...dysphagia:* American Speech-Language-Hearing Association: "Swallowing Disorders (Dysphagia) in Adults." http://www.asha.org/public/speech/swallowing/Swallowing Adults.htm

Castrogiovanni A: Communication facts: Special populations: Dysphagia–2008 edition. American Speech-Language-Hearing Association. http://www.asha.org/research/reports/dysphagia.htm

29. *Difficulty swallowing:* Wilkins T, Gillies RA, Thomas AM, Wagner PJ: The prevalence of dysphagia in primary care patients: A HamesNet research network study. *Journal of the American Board of Family Medicine* (2007) 20:144-50. http://www.jabfm.org/cgi/content/full/20/2/144?maxtoshow=&HITS=10&hits=10&RESULTFOR MAT=&author1=wilkins&fulltext=dysphagia&searchid=1&FIRSTIND EX=0&sortspec=relevance&resourcetype=HWCIT

30. *Swallowing problems can arise:* Logemann JA: "Introduction: Definitions and Basic Principles of Evaluation and Treatment of Swallowing Disorders" (Chapter 1), "Swallowing Disorders After Treatment for Oral and Oropharyngeal Cancer" (Chapter 7), "Swallowing Disorders After Treatment for Laryngeal Cancer" (Chapter 8), "Swallowing Disorders Caused by Neurologic Lesions from Which Some Recovery Can be Anticipated" (Chapter 9), "Swallowing Problems Associated with Degenerative Disease" (Chapter 10), in *Evaluation and Treatment of Swallowing Disorders, 2nd edition,* PRO-ED, Inc., Austin, TX, 1998, pp. 1-11, 251-79, 281-306, 307-28, 329-43.

30. *Neurologic refers to:* Carrau RL, Murry T: Pathophysiology of Swallowing Disorders. Part IV, in *Comprehensive Management of Swallowing Disorders,* Carrau RL, Murry T (eds.), Singular Publishing Group, Inc., San Diego, CA, 1999, pp. 91-233.

32. *Losing one's sense of smell or taste:* Carl LL, Johnson PR: "Medications Affecting Appetite, Taste, or Smell." Chapter 12, in

Notes

Drugs and Dysphagia: How Medications Can Affect Eating and Swallowing. PRO-ED, Inc., Austin, TX, 2006, pp. 219-36.

30. *Drug effect, or Sjögren's:* Brody JE: "When swallowing food becomes a problem." *New York Times*, July 20, 2004. http://www.nytimes.com/2004/07/20/health/personal-health-when-swallowing-food-becomes-a-problem.html?pagewanted=1

35. *Pulmonary Problems:* Gross RD, Atwood Jr CW, Ross SB, Olszewski JW, Eichhorn KA: The coordination of breathing and swallowing in chronic obstructive pulmonary disease. *American Journal of Respiratory and Critical Care Medicine* (2009) 179:559-65. http://ajrccm.atsjournals.org/cgi/content/abstract/179/7/559?maxtoshow=&HITS=10&hits=10&RESULTFORMAT=&searchid=1&FIRSTINDEX=0&minscore=5000&resourcetype=HWCIT

37. *Swallowing and Stroke:* Murry T, Carrau RL: "The Abnormal Swallow: Conditions and Diseases." Part III, in *Clinical Management of Swallowing Disorders, Second Edition.* Plural Publishing, Inc., San Diego, CA, 2006, p, 47.

38. *Because the swallowing reflex:* Gross RD, Atwood Jr CW, Ross SB, Eichhorn KA, Olszewski JW, Doyle PJ: The coordination of breathing and swallowing in Parkinson's disease. *Dysphagia* (2008) 23:136-45. http://www.springerlink.com/content/c8047346485t4312/

Martino R, Foley N, Bhogal S, Diamant N, Speechley M, Teasell R: Dysphagia after stroke: Incidence, diagnosis, and pulmonary complications. *Stroke* (2005) 36:2756-63. http://stroke.ahajournals.org/cgi/content/full/36/12/2756

40. *Favorite target of scleroderma:* Sheehan NJ: Dysphagia and other manifestations of oesophageal involvement in the musculoskeletal diseases. *Rheumatology* (2008) 47:746-52. http://rheumatology.oxfordjournals.org/cgi/reprint/ken029v1

40. *Stricture formation...cancer:* Enzinger PC, Mayer RJ: Esophageal cancer. *New England Journal of Medicine* (2003) 349:2241-52.

Chapter 4. What To Do About Choking

46. *Food, pills, or non-food objects:* Warshawsky ME: Foreign body aspiration. *eMedicine.* Updated Jan. 3, 2008. http://emedicine.medscape.com/article/298940-overview

47. *Adult male...trachea:* Breatnach E, Abbott GC, Fraser RB: Dimensions of the normal human trachea. *American Journal of Roentgenology* (1984) 141:903-06. http://www.ajronline.org/cgi/reprint/142/5/903.pdf

48. *The elderly are at highest risk:* Dolkas L, Stanley C, Smith AM, Vilke GM: Deaths associated with choking in San Diego County. *Journal of Forensic Sciences* (2007) 52:176-79.

Ekberg O, Feinberg M: Clinical and demographic data in 75 patients with near-fatal choking episodes. *Dysphagia* (1992) 7:205-08.

Mittelman RE, Wetli CV: The fatal café coronary: Foreign-body airway obstruction. *Journal of the American Medical Association* (1982) 247:1285-88.

48. *Missing teeth...dentures:* Wick R, Gilbert JD, Byard RW: Café coronary syndrome – Fatal choking on food: An autopsy approach. *Journal of Clinical Forensic Medicine* (2006) 13:135-38, 2006. http://www.ncbi.nlm.nih.gov/pubmed/16356749

48. *With Parkinson disease:* Gross RD, Atwood Jr CW, Ross SB, Eichhorn KA, Olszewski JW, Doyle PJ: The coordination of breathing and swallowing in Parkinson's disease. *Dysphagia* (2008) 23:136-45. http://www.springerlink.com/content/c8047346485t4312/

49. *A person choking on food:* Haugen RK: The café coronary: Sudden deaths in restaurants. *Journal of the American Medical Association* (1963) 186:142-43.

51. *Perform the Heimlich maneuver:* Heimlich HJ: Pop goes the café coronary. *Emergency Medicine* June 1974, 154-55.

Heimlich HJ: A Life-Saving Maneuver to Prevent Food-Choking. *Journal of the American Medical Association* (1975) 234:398-401.

Heimlich Institute: How to do the Heimlich maneuver. 2007. http://www.heimlichinstitute.org/page.php?id=34

MedlinePlus: Choking–adult or child over 1 year. Updated July 8, 2009. http://www.nlm.nih.gov/medlineplus/ency/article/000049.htm

56. *Some sources recommend:* American Red Cross: Choking Emergencies. 2008. http://american.redcross.org/site/PageNavigator/SafetyNET/April_08/chokingemergencies

Notes

56. *Of the American Heart:* American Heart Association: Heimlich Maneuver. AHA Recommendation, April 18, 2010. http://www.american heart.org/presenter.jhtml?identifier=4605

American Heart Association: Relief of Choking in Children, 10/28/2008. http://www.americanheart.org/presenter.jhtml?identifier=3025002

Day RL, Crelin ES, DuBois AB: Choking: The Heimlich abdominal thrust vs. back blows: An approach to measurement of inertial and aerodynamic forces. *Pediatrics* (1982) 70:113-19.

58. *As Dr. Henry Heimlich explained:* Albert Lasker Public Service Award: 1984 Winners. http://www.laskerfoundation.org/awards/1984public.htm

Chapter 5. Aspiration and Pneumonia

64. *Strictly speaking, aspiration:* Logemann JA: "Introduction: Definitions and Basic Principles of Evaluation and Treatment of Swallowing Disorders," Chapter 1 in *Evaluation and Treatment of Swallowing Disorders, 2nd edition*, PRO-ED, Inc., Austin, TX, 1998, p. 5.

64. *Aspiration can result:* Smith Hammond CA, Goldstein LB: Cough and aspiration of food and liquids due to oral-pharyngeal dysphagia. ACCP evidence-based clinical practice guidelines. *Chest* (2006) 129:154S-168S.

64. *Lack of coordination:* Gross RD, Atwood Jr CW, Ross SB, Olszewski JW, Eichhorn KA: The coordination of breathing and swallowing in chronic obstructive pulmonary disease. *American Journal of Respiratory and Critical Care Medicine* (2009) 179:559-65. http://ajrccm.atsjournals.org/cgi/content/abstract/179/7/559?maxtoshow=&HITS=10&hits=10&RESULTFORMAT=&searchid=1&FIRSTINDEX=0&minscore=5000&resourcetype=HWCIT

Martino R, Foley N, Bhogal S, Diamant N, Speechley M, Teasell R: Dysphagia after stroke: Incidence, diagnosis, and pulmonary complications. *Stroke* (2005) 36:2756-63. http://stroke.ahajournals.org/cgi/content/full/36/12/2756

67. *Aspiration pneumonia is:* Marik PE: Aspiration pneumonitis and aspiration pneumonia. *New England Journal of Medicine* (2001) 344:665-71.

Marik PE, Kaplan D: Aspiration pneumonia and dysphagia in the elderly. *Chest* (2003) 124:328-36. http://chestjournal.chestpubs.org/content/124/1/328.full.pdf+html

67. *Stomach acid...pneumonitis:* Falestiny MN, Yu VL: "Aspiration Pneumonia," Chapter 55 in *Comprehensive Management of Swallowing Disorders*, Carrau RL, Murry T (eds.), Singular Publishing Group, Inc., San Diego, CA, 1999, pp. 383-87.

Marks JW: Gastroesophageal reflux disease (GERD, acid reflux, heartburn). MedicineNet.com http://www.medicinenet.com/gastroesophageal_reflux_disease_gerd/article.htm

68. *Chronic cough, unexplaind pneumonia:* Morehead RS: Gastro-oesophageal reflux disease and non-asthma lung disease. *European Respiratory Review* (2009) 18:233-43. http://err.ersjournals.com/cgi/content/full/18/114/233

68. *An Unsettling Fact:* Ramsey D, Smithard D, Kalra L: Silent aspiration: What do we know? *Dysphagia* (2005) 20:218-25.

Ramsey DJC, Smithard DG, Kalra L: Early Assessments of dysphagia and aspiration risk in acute stroke patients. *Stroke* (2003) 34:1252-57. http://stroke.ahajournals.org/cgi/reprint/34/5/1252

Smith Hammond CA, Goldstein LB: Cough and aspiration of food and liquids due to oral-pharyngeal dysphagia: ACCP evidence-based clinical practice guidelines. *Chest* (2006) 129:154S-168S. http://chestjournal.chestpubs.org/content/129/1_suppl/154S.full.pdf+html

68. *Silent aspiration can occur:* Huxley EJ, Viroslav J, Gray WR, Pierce AK: Pharyngeal aspiration in normal adults and patients with depressed consciousness. *American Journal of Medicine* (1978) 64:564-68.

Chapter 6. Medication: A Double-Edged Sword

74. *Life. But their side effects:* Alvi A: "Iatrogenic swallowing disorders: Medications." Chapter 17 in *Comprehensive Management of Swallowing Disorders*, Carrau RL, Murry T (eds.), Singular Publishing Group, Inc., San Diego, CA 1999, pp. 119-124.

Notes

74. *When...multiple medications:* Gorard DA: Escalating polypharmacy. *Quarterly Journal of Medicine* (2006) 99:797-800. http://qjmed.oxfordjournals.org/cgi/reprint/99/11/797

Carl L, Johnson P: Drugs and dysphagia. *Perspectives on Swallowing and Swallowing Disorders (Dysphagia)* (2008) 17:143-48.

74. *Multiple medications:* Hajjar ER, Cafiero AC, Hanlon JT: Polypharmacy in elderly patients. *American Journal of Geriatric Pharmacotherapy* (2007) 5:345-51.

74. *Greater likelihood of...error:* Goulding MR: Inappropriate medication prescribing for elderly ambulatory care patients. *Archives of Internal Medicine* (2004) 164:305-12. http://archinte. ama-assn.org/cgi/reprint/164/3/305

75. *In the brain, acetylcholine:* Ancelin ML, Artero S, Portet F, Dupuy A-M, Touchon J, Ritchie K: Non-degenerative mild cognitive impairment in elderly people and use of anticholinergic drugs: longitudinal cohort study. *British Medical Journal* (2006) 332:455-59. http://www.bmj.com/cgi/content/abstract/bmj.38740.439664.DEv1

79. *Be on the alert:* Mintzer J, Burns A: Anticholinergic side-effects of drugs in elderly people. *Journal of the Royal Society of Medicine* (2000) 93:457-62.

79. *Sense of smell:* Carl LL, Johnson PR: "Medications Affecting Appetite, Taste, or Smell." Chapter 12, in *Drugs and Dysphagia: How Medications Can Affect Eating and Swallowing.* PRO-ED, Inc., Austin, TX, 2006, pp. 219-36.

80. *Muscle movement:* Ruschena D, Mullen PE, Palmer S, Burgess P, Cordner SM, Drummer OH, Wallace C, Barry-Walsh J: Choking deaths: The role of antipsychotic medication. *British Journal of Psychiatry* (2003) 183:446-50.

80. *Microenvironment:* Agarwala SS, Sbeitan I: "Iatrogenic Swallowing Disorders: Chemotherapy." Chapter 18 in *Comprehensive Management of Swallowing Disorders*, Carrau RL, Murry T (eds.), Singular Publishing Group, Inc., San Diego, CA 1999, pp. 124-29.

80. *The esophagus is exquisitely vulnerable:* Carl LL, Johnson PR: "Medications That Cause Esophageal Injury," in *Drugs and Dysphagia: How Medications Can Affect Eating and Swallowing.* PRO-ED, Inc., Austin, TX, 2006, pp. 261-62.

Jaspersen D: Drug-induced oesophageal disorders: Pathogenesis, incidence, prevention and management. *Drug Safety* (2000) 22:237-49. http://www.ncbi.nlm.nih.gov/pubmed/10738847

81. *Some medications cause...esophageal:* Lagergren J, Bergstrom R, Adami H-O, Nyren O: Association between medications that relax the lower esophageal sphincter and risk for esophageal adencarcinoma. *Annals of Internal Medicine* (2000) 133:165-75.

82. *Use your favorite search engine:* MedlinePlus: Drugs, Supplements, and Herbal Information. U.S. National Library of Medicine and National Institutes of Health, Department of Health and Human Services. http://www.nlm.nih.gov/medlineplus/druginformation.html

U.S. Food and Drug Administration, U.S. Department of Health and Human Services. http://www.fda.gov/Drugs/default.htm

86. *When....emotionally-based:* Chatoor I, Conley C, Dickson L. Food refusal after an incident of choking: A posttraumatic eating disorder. *Journal of the American Academy of Child and Adolescent Psychiatry* (1988) 27:105-10. http://download.journals.elsevierhealth.com/pdfs/journals/0890-8567/PIIS0890856709653624.pdf

Shapiro J, Franko DL, Gagne A: Phagophobia: A form of psychogenic dysphagia. A new entity. *Annals of Otology, Rhinology and Laryngology* (1997) 106:286-90.

Chapter 7. Treating Swallowing Problems

91. *Treatment....individually-tailored:* Carrau RL, Murry T: "Nonsurgical Treatment of Swallowing Disorders" (Chapters 34-37) and "Surgical Treatment of Swallowing Disorders" (Chapters 38-50) in *Comprehensive Management of Swallowing Disorders*, Carrau RL, Murry T (eds.), Singular Publishing Group, Inc. San Diego, CA,1999, pp. 235-62, 263-343.

Logemann JA: "Management of the Patient with Oropharyngeal Swallowing Disorders." Chapter 6 in *Evaluation and Treatment of Swallowing Disorders, 2nd edition*, PRO-ED, Inc., Austin, TX, 1998, pp. 191-250.

Notes

Palmer JL, Metheny NA: Preventing aspiration in older adults with dysphagia. *American Journal of Nursing* (2008) 108:40-48. http://www.nursingcenter.com/library/JournalArticle.asp?Article_ID=770844

Smith Hammond CA, Goldstein LB: Cough and aspiration of food and liquids due to oral-pharyngeal dysphagia: ACCP evidence-based clinical practice guidelines. *Chest* (2006) 129:154S-168S. http://chestjournal.chestpubs.org/content/129/1_suppl/154S.full.pdf +html

96. *Mealtime Strategies:* Lieberman A, McCall M: *100 Questions & Answers About Parkinson Disease.* Jones and Bartlett Publishers, Sudbury, MA, 2003, pp. 123-27, 158-61.

Schwarz SP: Eating and drinking tips for people with swallowing difficulties. In Chapter 8 in *Parkinson's Disease: 300 Tips for Making Life Easier, Second Edition.* Demos Medical Publishing, LLC, New York, NY, 2006, pp. 66-72.

99. *Modification of the diet:* Logemann JA: Oropharyngeal dysphagia and nutritional management. *Current Opinion in Clinical Nutrition and Metabolic Care* (2007) 10:611-14.

Carnaby G, Hankey GJ, Pizzi J: Behavioural intervention for dysphagia in acute stroke: A randomised controlled trial. *Lancet Neurology* (2006) 5:31-37. http://www.ncbi.nlm.nih.gov/pubmed/16361020

99. *Drinks....thickening agent:* Logemann JA, Gensler G, Robbins J, Lindblad AS, Brandt D, Hind JA, Kosek S, Dikeman K, Kazandjian M, Gramigna GD, Lundy D, McGarvey-Toler S, Miller Gardner PJ: A randomized study of three interventions for aspiration of thin liquids in patients with dementia or Parkinson's disease. *Journal of Speech, Language, and Hearing Research* (2008) 51:173-83. http://jslhr.asha.org/cgi/reprint/51/1/173

101. *For those....modified diet:* Achilles E: *The Dysphagia Cookbook. Great Tasting and Nutritious Recipes for People with Swallowing Difficulties.* Cumberland House. Nashville, TN, 2004.

Weihoffen DL, Robbins J, Sullivan PA: *Easy-to-Swallow, Easy-to-Chew Cookbook. Over 150 Tasty and Nutritious Recipes for People Who Have Difficulty Swallowing.* John Wiley and Sons, NY, 2002.

101. *Common maneuver....chin tuck:* Ashford J, McCabe D, Wheeler-Hegland K, Frymark T, Mullen R, Musson N, Schooling T, Smith

Hammond C: Evidence-based systematic review: Oropharyngeal dysphagia behavioral treatments. Part III-Impact of dysphagia treatments on populations with neurological disorders. *Journal of Rehabilitation Research and Development* (2009) 46:195-204. http://www.rehab.research.va.gov/jour/09/46/2/pdf/ashford.pdf

101. *Keep in mind that....eye contact:* Gawande A: "The way we age now." In *Annals of Medicine: The New Yorker*, April 30, 2007. http://www.newyorker.com/reporting/2007/04/30/070430fa_fact_gawande

101. *The therapist....effortful swallow:* Wheeler-Hegland K, Ashford J, Frymark T, McCabe D, Mullen R, Musson N, Smith Hammond C: Schooling T: Evidence-based systematic review: Oropharyngeal dysphagia behavioral treatments. Part II-Impact of dysphagia treatment on normal swallow function. *Journal of Rehabilitation Research and Development* (2009) 46:185-94. http://www.rehab.research.va.gov/jour/09/46/2/pdf/page185.pdf

101. *Exercises for Swallowing:* Robbins J, Kays SA, Gangnon RE, Hind JA, Hewitt AL, Gentry LR, Taylor AJ: The effects of lingual exercise in stroke patients with dysphagia. *Archives of Physical Medicine and Rehabilitation* (2007) 88:150-58.

102. *Even the upper esophageal:* Shaker R, Antonik S: The Shaker exercise. *US Gastroenterology Review* (2006) 2:19-20. http://www.touchgastroenterology.com/articles/shaker-exercise For a video of the Shaker exercise, see http://www.mcw.edu/display/docid26360.htm

102. *Motivation...cognitive limitations:* Logemann J, Sonies B: Grand rounds: Dysphagia. *The ASHA Leader* July 20, 2004. http://www.asha.org/Publications/leader/2004/040720/f040720a.htm

103. *To enhance the sensory:* Miller AJ: Neuroscience of swallowing: Strategies in rehabilitation. *Perspectives on Swallowing and Swallowing Disorders (Dysphagia)* (2008) 17:121-27. http://div13perspectives.asha.org/cgi/reprint/17/4/121

103. *Stimulation....by means of electrodes:* Carnaby-Mann GD, Crary MA: Examining the evidence on neuromuscular electrical stimulation for swallowing. *Archives of Otolaryngology—Head and Neck Surgery* (2007) 133:564-71.

Notes

Ludlow C: Electrical stimulation and dysphagia: What we do and don't know. *The ASHA Leader* 13(3), 8-11, March 4, 2008. http://www.asha.org/Publications/leader/2008/080304/f080304a/

105. *Oral Care Counts:* Ashford JR, Skelley M: Oral care and the elderly. *Perspectives on Swallowing and Swallowing Disorders (Dysphagia)* (2008) 17:19-26. http://div13perspectives.asha.org/cgi/content/full/17/1/19

Mojon P: Oral health and respiratory infection. *Journal of the Canadian Dental Association* (2002) 68:340-05.

106. *Another thing you can do:* Medina-Walpole AM, Katz PR: Nursing home-acquired pneumonia. *Journal of the American Geriatrics Society* (1999) 47:1005-15.

Chapter 8. Getting Help

113. *Settings...include hospitals:* Weindling F-H: Speech-language pathology: A home care viewpoint. *American Journal of Speech-Language Pathology* (2000) 9:99-106.

113. *Examination of Swallowing:* Doggett DL, Tappe KA, Mitchell MD, Chapell R, Coates V, Turkelson CM: Prevention of pneumonia in elderly stroke patients by systematic diagnosis and treatment of dysphagia: An evidence-based comprehensive analysis of the literature. *Dysphagia* (2001) 16:279-95.

Hinchey JA, Shephard T, Furie K, Smith D, Wang D, Tonn S: Formal dysphagia screening protocols prevent pneumonia. *Stroke* (2005) 36:1972-76. http://stroke.ahajournals.org/cgi/reprint/36/9/1972

Ramsey DJC, Smithard DG, Kalra L: Early assessments of dysphagia and aspiration risk in acute stroke patients. *Stroke* (2003) 34:1252-57. http://stroke.ahajournals.org/cgi/reprint/34/5/1252

American Speech-Language-Hearing Association. Scope of practice in speech-language pathology. Rockville, MD. 2001. http://www.nslha.org/media/Scope_of_Practice_SLP.pdf

116. *Include...oxygen saturation:* Westergren A: Detection of eating difficulties after stroke: A systematic review. *International Nursing Review* (2006) 53:143-49.

117. *The modified barium swallow:* Logemann J: "Videofluoroscopy" (pp. 58-61) and "Videofluoroscopic procedure—The modified barium swallow" (pp. 168-85) In *Evaluation and Treatment of Swallowing Disorders, 2nd edition,* PRO-ED, Inc., Austin, TX, 1998.

118. *Fiberoptic endoscopic evaluation:* Logemann J: Videoendoscopy. In *Evaluation and Treatment of Swallowing Disorders, 2nd edition,* PRO-ED, Inc., Austin, TX, 1998, pp. 54-59.

Murry T, Carrau RL: "Functional Tests of Swallowing." Chapter 12 in *Comprehensive Management of Swallowing Disorders,* Carrau RL, Murry T (eds.), Singular Publishing Group, Inc., San Diego, CA, 1999, pp. 75-79.

118. *In addition to a speech-language pathologist:* Logemann JA: "Multidisciplinary Management of Dysphagia." Chapter 13 in *Evaluation and Treatment of Swallowing Disorders, 2nd edition,* PRO-ED, Inc., Austin, TX, 1998, pp. 367-73.

119. *Swallowing is so closely related:* American Speech-Language-Hearing Association: End-of-life issues in speech-language pathology. http://www.asha.org/slp/clinical/endoflife.htm#Top and http://www.asha.org/slp/EOLresources.htm

Landes TL: Ethical issues involved in patients' rights to refuse artificially administered nutrition and hydration and implications for the speech-language pathologist. *American Journal of Speech-Language Pathology* (1999) 8:109-17. http://ajslp.asha.org/cgi/reprint/8/2/109?maxtoshow=&HITS=10&hits=10&RESULTFORMAT=&searchid=1&FIRSTINDEX=0&sortspec=relevance&volume=8&firstpage=109&resourcetype=HWCIT

119. *May relate to tube-feeding:* Casarett D, Kapo J, Caplan A: Appropriate use of artificial nutrition and hydration—Fundamental principles and recommendations. *New England Journal of Medicine* (2005) 353:2607-12.

Mitchell SL: A 93-year-old man with advanced dementia and eating problems. *Journal of the American Medical Association* (2007) 298:2527-36. http://jama.ama-assn.org/cgi/content/full/298/21/2527

Morrison RS, Meier DE: Palliative care. *New England Journal of Medicine* (2004) 350:2582-90.

Vollman J, Burke WJ, Kupfer RY, Tessler S, Friedel DM, Ozick LA, Gillick M: Rethinking the role of tube feeding in patients with advanced dementia. *New England Journal of Medicine* (2000) 342:206-10.

120. *A patient who rejects:* Sharp HM, Bryant KN: Ethical issues in dysphagia: When patients refuse assessment or treatment. *Seminars in Speech and Language* (2003) 24:285-99.

121. *An Advance Directive:* Mueller PS, Hook CC, Fleming KC: Ethical issues in geriatrics: A guide for clinicians. *Mayo Clinic Proceedings* (2004) 79:554-62. http://www.mayoclinicproceedings. com/content/79/4/554.long

121. *It is your love that guides:* Ostwald SK, Davis S, Hersch G, Kelley C, Godwin KM: Evidence-based educational guidelines for stroke survivors after discharge home. *Journal of Neuroscience Nursing* (2008) 40:173-91. http://www.ncbi.nlm.nih.gov/pmc/ articles/PMC2743441/pdf/nihms-107369.pdf

Chapter 9. Mindful Swallowing

126. *If you are mindful while eating:* Bays JC: *Mindful Eating: A Guide to Rediscovering a Healthy and Joyful Relationship with Food.* Shambhala Press, Boston, MA, 2009.

Somov, PG: *Eating the Moment: 141 Mindful Practices To Overcome Overeating One Meal at a Time.* New Harbinger Publications, Oakland, CA, 2008.

ADDITIONAL READINGS

Avadian B: *"Where's My Shoes?": My Father's Walk Through Alzheimer's, Second Edition*. North Star Books, Pearblossom, CA, 2005.

Coskie DF-S: *Unthinkable: A Mother's Tragedy, Terror, and Triumph through a Child's Traumatic Brain Injury*. Wyatt-MacKenzie Publishing, Deadwood, OR, 2010.

Graboys T, Zheutlin P: *Life in the Balance. A Physician's Memoir of Life, Love, and Loss with Parkinson's Disease and Dementia*. Union Square Press, New York, NY, 2008.

Mace N, Rabins P: *The 36-Hour Day: A Family Guide to Caring for Persons with Alzheimer's Disease, Related Dementing Illnesses, and Memory Loss in Later Life, Fourth Edition*. Warner Books, New York, NY, 2006.

Marcell J: *Elder Rage—or, Take My Father...Please! How To Survive Caring For Aging Parents*. Impressive Press, Irvine, CA, 2001.

Martensen R: *A Life Worth Living: A Doctor's Reflections on Illness in a High-Tech Era*. Farrar, Strauss and Giroux, New York, NY, 2008.

McCullough D: *My Mother, Your Mother: Embracing "Slow Medicine"—The Compassionate Approach to Caring For Your Aging Loved Ones*. HarperCollins Publishers, New York, NY, 2008.

165

Meyer MM, Derr P: *The Comfort of Home, 3rd Edition. A Complete Guide for Caregivers*. CareTrust Publications, Portland, OR, 2007.

Northrup C: *Mother-Daughter Wisdom: Understanding the Crucial Link Between Mothers, Daughters, and Health*. Random House Publishing Group, New York, NY, 2006.

Panther K: The Frazier Water Protocol. *Swallowing and Swallowing Disorders*, March 2005. http://www.slpnetwork.org/archives/Meeting%2011-06-08/Frazier%20Protocol.pdf

Schwarz SP: *Multiple Sclerosis: 300 Tips for Making Life Easier, Second Edition*. Demos Medical Publishing, New York, NY, 2006.

Seuss D: *You're Only Old Once!* Random House, Inc., New York, NY, 1986.

Span P: *When the Time Comes: Families with Aging Parents Share their Struggles and Solutions*. Springboard Press, New York, NY, 2009.

Winakur J: *Memory Lessons: A Doctor's Story*. Hyperion, New York, NY, 2009.

RESOURCES

Alzheimer Disease

Alzheimer's Association
www.alz.org
(800) 272-3900

Alzheimer's Disease
Education and Referral
Center (ADEAR), U.S.
National Institutes of
Health, National
Institute on Aging
http://www.nia.nih.gov/
alzheimers
(800) 438-4380

Alzheimer's Foundation
of America
www.alzfdn.org
(866) 232-8484

Alzheimer Society
of Canada
www.alzheimer.ca
(416) 488-8722

Blogs

The Caregiver's Voice
www.thecaregiversvoice.com

The New Old Age:
Caring and Coping
The New York Times
http://newoldage.blogs.
nytimes.com/

Transition Aging Parents
www.transitionagingparents
.com

Caregiving

American Association of
Homes and Services
for the Aging
www.aahsa.org
(202) 783-2242

American Association of
Retired Persons (AARP)
www.aarp.org
(800) 424-3410

Caregiver.com
www.caregiver.com
(800) 829-2734

Eldercare Locator
www.eldercare.gov
(800) 677-1116

167

Family Caregiver Alliance
www.caregiver.org
(800) 445-8106

National Alliance
for Caregiving
www.caregiving.org
info@caregiving.org

National Council on Aging
www.ncoa.org
(202) 479-1200

National Family Caregivers
Association
www.nfcacares.org
(301) 942-6430

Legal

National Academy of
Elder Law Attorneys
www.naela.com
(703) 942-5711

National Senior Citizen's
Law Center
www.nsclc.org
(202) 289-6976

Multiple Sclerosis

Montel Williams
MS Foundation
www.montelms.org
info@montelms.org

Multiple Sclerosis
Association of America
www.msassociation.org
(800) 532-7667

Multiple Sclerosis
Foundation
www.msfocus.org
(888) 673-6287

National Multiple
Sclerosis Society
www.nationalmssociety.org
(800) 344-4867

Parkinson Disease

American Parkinson
Disease Association
www.apdaparkinson.org
(800) 223-2732

Michael J. Fox Foundation
for Parkinson Research
www.michaeljfox.org
(800) 708-7644

National Parkinson
Foundation
www.parkinson.org
(800) 327-4545

Parkinson's Disease
Foundation
www.pdf.org
(800) 457-6676

Resources

Stroke

American Stroke
Association
www.StrokeAssociation.org
(888) 478-7653

Heart and Stroke
Foundation of Canada
ww2.heartandstroke.ca
/splash/
(613) 569-4361

National Institute of
Neurological Disorders
and Stroke
www.ninds.nih.gov

National Stroke
Association
www.stroke.org
(800) 787-6537

Additional Resources

ALS Association
www.alsa.org
(818) 880-9007

American Autoimmune
Related Disease
Association
www.aarda.org
(800) 598-4668

American Cancer Society
www.cancer.org
(800) 227-2345

American Society on Aging
www.asaging.org
(800) 537-9728

American Speech-
Language-Hearing
Association (ASHA)
www.asha.org
(800) 638-8255

Brain Injury Association
of America
www.biausa.org
(703) 761-0750

Head Injury Association
www.lihia.org
(631) 543-2245

Huntington's Disease
Society of America
www.hdsa.org
(800) 345-4372

Meeting Life's Challenges
www.meetinglifeschallenges
.com
(608) 824-0402

Muscular Dystrophy
Association
www.mda.org

Myasthenia Gravis
Foundation of America
www.myasthenia.org
(800) 541-5454

National Hospice
and Palliative Care
Organization
www.nhpco.org
(703) 837-1500

PubMed Central,
U.S. National Institutes
of Health.
www.ncbi.nlm.nih.gov/pmc

Solutions For Better Aging
www.AgeNet.com
(888) 405-4242

United States
Administration on Aging
www.aoa.gov
(202) 619-0724

Wilson Disease
Association
www.wilsonsdisease.org
(888) 264-1450

INDEX

A

abdominal thrusts. *See*
  Heimlich maneuver
acetylcholine, 75
achalasia, 40, 41
advance directive, 107, 121
alcohol, 35, 48-49, 70, 121
ALS. *See* amyotrophic lateral
  sclerosis
Alzheimer disease, 6, 7, 32-
  33, 64, 66, 102
amyotrophic lateral
  sclerosis, 6, 10, 30, 33,
  36, 38, 64, 66
anticholinergic drugs, 75-79,
  82, 143-45
  listed, 78, 143-45
  side effects, 75-79
  therapeutic effects, 76
anxiety, 5, 29, 45, 52, 74, 79,
  98, 121
  choking and, 52
  mouth-breathing and, 35, 98
  pill-taking, 86, 88
ASHA (American Speech-
  Language-Hearing
  Association), 113

aspiration, 4, 18, 29, 36, 39,
  56, 63-70, 91, 94, 96, 99,
  100, 103-06, 116, 119-20,
  122, 126
  causes of, 35, 41
  chest x-rays and, 116, 118
  definition, 63
  foods of mixed
    consistency and, 94-96
  illustration, 65
  overview, 70
  oxygen saturation and, 116
  penetration vs., 64
  pneumonia and, 4, 67-68,
    119
  pneumonitis after, 67-68
  silent, 66, 68-69
  symptoms suggesting, 66
  tearing and, 66, 68, 70, 98
  tests for, 115-18
  tube-feeding and, 69, 104,
    119, 121
  voice change and, 30, 58, 66,
    68, 69, 70, 111, 115, 131
  vomiting and, 67
  wheezing and, 66, 68, 69,
    70, 114, 131
  Zenker diverticulum and, 39

Index

Index

Index

illustrations, 16, 19-20, 23
phenothiazines, 80, 144
pills, 29, 46, 73-88, 122, 138-39
    anxiety with, 86,88
    problems with, 82-83
    specialized cups, 87-88, 98
    tips for swallowing, 82-83,
        138-39
pneumonia, 4, 6-7, 35, 40, 58,
    63-70, 99, 104, 106, 119-20,
    122
    aspiration causing, 4, 63-70,
        104-05, 116, 126
    bacterial, 35, 105
    chemical, 40
    after choking, 58
    illustration, 65
    prevention, 70, 93
    recurrent, 66
    symptoms, 68
    tube-feeding and, 104
pneumonitis, 67-68, 70
pocketing, 18, 83, 97
POPE, 15
positioning, 26, 93-94, 106,
    118, 137
prevention, 3, 10, 56, 59, 70,
    100, 104, 106, 125, 140
prostheses, 104

Q

quality-of-life issues. *See*
    decisions

R

radiotherapy, 32, 34
reflex, swallowing. *See*
    swallowing reflex
reflux, gastroesophageal, 40,
    73, 80-81, 87, 94, 140
regurgitation,
    achalasia and, 40
    nasal, 30, 38, 98, 104, 131
    scleroderma and, 40
    Zenker diverticulum and, 39
runny nose, 29, 66, 131, 138

S

safe swallowing suggestions,
    106, 137-40
safety net, 21, 38
saliva, 7, 15-17, 24-25, 32-33,
    36, 41, 64, 73, 75, 77, 79, 83,
    86, 88, 96, 104-05, 137, 139
    lack of, 41, 64, 73, 77, 79, 88.
    See also anticholinergic
    drugs
scleroderma, 40
sensory stimulation, 103
side effects. *See* drugs;
    medication
silent aspiration, 66, 68-69
Sjögren's syndrome, 32
smell, sense of, 15, 17, 32,
    41, 73, 79, 92, 127
    loss of, 32, 41, 73, 79, 92
soft palate, 16, 19-21, 23, 38,
    64,104, 115

Index

V

vaccine, pneumococcal, 93, 106
videofluoroscopic swallowing study. *See* barium swallow, modified
vision, blurred, 75-77, 82
  See also drugs, anticholinergic
vocal cords, 21, 38, 64
voice, change in,
  aspiration and, 30, 66, 68-70, 111, 115, 131
  choking and, 50, 58
  gargly, 66, 131
  nasal, 38, 131
vomiting, 22, 34, 67
  aspiration and, 67
  dehydration and, 34
  pneumonitis and, 67

W

walk-through, swallowing, 24
weakness, 4, 31, 33, 35, 38, 41, 68, 97, 112
wheezing, 50, 66, 68-70, 114, 131, 139
Wilson disease, 34, 36
wrong tube, 63, 70

X

x-rays,
  chest, 116, 118
  modified barium swallow, 117

Y

yeast infection, 34, 80, 114
Your Swallowing Story, 10, 147

Z

Zenker diverticulum, 39, 105

BOOK ORDER FORM

Order online through www.swallowsafely.com

By mail, please provide the information below and send check
or money order to

Inside/Outside Press
P.O. Box 661
Natick, MA 01760

I would like to order _____ books.   Price: $14.95 each.

MA residents: Please add $1.05 per book.

Shipping: Continental US add $4.00 for first book,

$2.00 for each additional book.

For Bulk Orders or Questions: swallowsafely@aol.com

Total_____

Shipping Address:

Name_____

Address_____ Apt. _____

City_____ State_____ Zip_____

Telephone_____E-mail_____

Would you like an autographed copy?   Yes   No

Would you like a copy of the book sent as a gift?

To whom?

Name_____

Address_____ Apt. _____

City_____ State_____ Zip_____